CW00556211

Every
you need to
know about
Colloidal Silver

- How to make it
- How to use it
- What it can do for you
- Costs involved
- Diseases it can heal
- Germs it can kill
- Testimonials
- Other interesting health facts

Max Crarer

ZEALAND PUBLISHING HOUSE LTD
Private Bag 12029, Tauranga. New Zealand.

First published 2000 by Max Crarer, Wairoa, New Zealand.
2nd Edition 2003 Revised and updated by David Coory at the written request of Max Crarer prior to his death in 2001.
Reprinted Oct 2006 minor revisions.
Reprinted Oct 2008 minor revisions.
Reprinted Nov 2009 minor revisions.
Reprinted Feb 2013 minor revisions
Kindle Version Feb 2013 minor revisions.

Further copies of this book can be obtained by contacting:

Zealand Publishing House Ltd
Private Bag 12029, Tauranga.
New Zealand.

Or by phone, fax, or internet (credit card required).

Phone 0800 140-141 (NZ only) or International +64 7 520-8103
Fax 0800 140-142 (NZ only) or International +64 7 543-0493

Internet www.zealandpublishing.co.nz
www.amazon.com

ISBN 9780987661777

The information and advice in this book is given in good faith and is not intended to replace competent medical advice.

Contents

3

PART TWO OF THIS BOOK

About this book

In reading this book you may decide I have no appreciation for the medical profession. This is not so. The profession is regarded by most people as a panacea for all ailments, which it can never be.

And because of strict 'union rules' within the profession, any doctor who discovers that natural remedies are far safer than any medical drug, or that minerals, vitamins, enzymes and amino acids are vital to good health, and tries to treat people by such methods, soon finds the door blocked by the power of drug monopolies and medical peer pressure.

Also, we have politicians who will grant millions of dollars for drugs that temporarily alleviate symptoms rather than actually heal a condition. These same politicians will not save a dollar of the taxpayer's money by allowing the writing of prescriptions for far cheaper natural healing substances. And the bulk of the powerful 'medical union' members throw their support behind the status quo.

No more glaring example of this can be found than in the use of Colloidal Silver, a product most doctors refuse to acknowledge, or in their ignorance do not even know exists.

Colloidal Silver could save much suffering and many lives, and the health service which is funded by we the taxpayers, millions of dollars every year.

Doctors who start life with the noble aim of helping people recover and stay healthy, must be quickly disillusioned by about two thirds of the population who believe they can indulge in any substance of abuse imaginable. Be it flooding their bodies with nicotine or alcohol, sniffing glue, taking drugs, spraying substances on their skin to stop the body ridding itself of poisons through sweat glands, eating unnatural substances like margarine, or gorging with sugar and fat-laden foods daily, so that some wander about like land-bound walruses.

Most people want a quick fix without in any way changing their living or eating habits. It's just not possible. Such people cannot ever live without a fortnightly visit to their doctor or chemist for medical drugs, mainly symptom palliatives which rarely heal.

All of us need doctors and surgeons to repair broken bones or bodies in case of accidents, or birth deformities, etc. But anyone with any intelligence should realise its not possible for a decreasing number of people, who produce wealth and pay taxes, to support an ever increasing number of people who deliberately make themselves and their children sick, and then expect doctors and the taxpayers to look after them.

THIS BOOK IS FOR THE 10% WHO CAN LOOK AFTER THEMSELVES!

It is for people who will use doctors to diagnose a problem and then, in most cases, treat themselves using the latest scientific knowledge and procedures. Procedures that are non invasive and require no use of drugs whatever.

You will also read later in this book of procedures that have been granted medical patents in the USA after overwhelming proofs have been supplied to the Patent Office. Procedures that will give you real hope if you suffer from Cancer, Hepatitis, Lupus, Aids, Epstein Barr, Influenza and many other so called 'incurable diseases.'

DO NOT READ THIS BOOK IF YOU ARE ADDICTED TO MEDICAL DRUGS, TOBACCO OR ALCOHOL. BECAUSE UNLESS AND UNTIL YOU ARE FREE OF THOSE ADDICTIONS, YOU CANNOT HELP YOURSELF OR BE HELPED. YOU MAY AS WELL STICK TO YOUR DOCTOR.

Finally, Good luck and good health. Sometimes they go together. Sometimes you can create your own.

MAX CRARER, May 2000.

What is Colloidal Silver?

Colloidal Silver is the most powerful, natural, anti-bacterial, anti-fungal, anti-viral, anti-parasite and body normalising substance ever discovered and used in medicine.

In laboratory tests, at just five parts per million, single-celled organisms such as bacteria, fungus and viruses are killed in just four or five minutes in its presence.

Dr Henry Crooks in his book **"Use of Colloids in Health and Disease"** states, *"There is no microbe known that is not killed by Colloidal Silver in six minutes or less, in a dilution as little as five parts per million."*

It is tasteless or almost so, odourless, non toxic. It has never been known to interact with any medical drug, or in normal doses to upset the stomach. In fact it is an aid to digestion.

Has anyone ever died through drinking or using Colloidal Silver?

No, there has never been a recorded case of anyone ever dying from using it internally or externally.

This is not surprising as the US Poison Control Centre gives a 'No Toxicity' rating for Colloidal Silver. In fact harmlessness is one of the cardinal attributes of colloids.

A healthy body must have an adequate intake of Silver in a colloid state to properly maintain the immune system.

What is a colloid?

A colloid is a liquid containing tiny particles of any kind of mineral, little larger than atoms. In this state colloids are the smallest particle of a mineral that can exist and retain its own identifying characteristic.

It is possible to create colloids of any mineral. Sea water contains colloids of all minerals. They are so tiny that they are permanently suspended in the water. It has been estimated that the sea contains around 8000 million tons of colloidal gold.

Are colloids essential to life?

Indeed, colloids of many minerals are absolutely essential to all life. Healthy animal and plant life cannot exist without a reasonable supply of colloidal minerals. Lack of essential colloids leads to chronic ill health among both animals and plants.

We humans often ingest colloids of various poisonous minerals. Even swallowing sea water will do that. But because they are colloids our bodies can easily deal with them. They cast them out as unneeded wastes, just as they do with excess vitamins.

Fruit and vegetable juices are rich in colloids and are an excellent way to preserve bodily health.

Why should we treat ourselves with Colloidal Silver?

Two good reasons.

First, it is the most powerful all-purpose antibiotic and healer ever discovered.

Second, it is the cheapest antibiotic to use and make. It acts against some 650 pathogens (disease organisms) in one operation, with no side effects whatsoever.

How old do you need to be to use it?

Any age; from newly conceived embryos, pregnant mothers, new-born infants, children, to an oldster dying of cancer.

What part of the body can it be used on?

Any part where you can possibly place it. Inside the body by swallowing. In the ears or eyes with a sprayer or dropper. On any external part of the body by spraying or on a soaked pad, or as a gel. In the lungs with a nebuliser. In the bowel with an enema, or in the vagina with a syringe. Even in the blood by injection in an emergency.

Does it sting?

No, not even in a new-born baby's eyes.

Is it possible to overdose on Colloidal Silver?

You can overdose on many supposedly harmless things and possibly kill yourself. Try eating a cup of salt, or a bag of sugar!

Unless you went on an impossible 'binge' of Colloidal Silver it should only do you good. The normal maximum

10

recommended dose is 2 teaspoons (10 ml) daily of 5 ppm strength.

For experimental purposes I personally drink a small glassful daily, around 180 mls, and have done so with no ill effects for over a year. On the contrary I have experienced only beneficial results.

Because it is in a colloidal state (or ionised) Colloidal Silver is absorbed in the mouth, throat and stomach. Therefore it does not harm friendly bacteria or enzymes in the intestines.

I have read of an experimenter in 1985 who drank one litre of high strength Colloidal Silver for several weeks. He did not eat Acidophilus yoghurt to compensate in any way for a possible kill of friendly intestinal bacteria. He stated that the only side effect was that he *"seemed to feel healthier and had no colds or aches."*

Can Colloidal Silver be injected intravenously?

Yes, it was being used with remarkable results over 80 years ago.

Colloidal Silver commonly used in 1919

No, that's not a misprint! Colloidal Silver was well known in 1919. The founder of a worldwide pharmaceutical company Alfred Searle wrote, *"Applying Colloidal Silver to human subjects has been done in a large number of cases with astonishingly successful results. For internal administration, orally or hypodermically, it has the advantage of being fatal to parasites without toxic action on its host. It is quite stable. It protects rabbits from ten times the lethal dose of Tetanus or Diphtheria toxin."*

What is Silver?

Silver is what is known as a heavy metal. It is almost white, and strongly reflects light. It is a very durable metal, and like gold it can be beaten into extremely thin sheets.

One ounce of silver can be beaten into an unflawed sheet of about 10 square metres, or for us oldies who don't deal in square metres, that's over 100 square feet. This knowledge has been with us for thousands of years. But it is only in the past couple of centuries in the western world that Silver has been used for anything else but art, cutlery, kitchenware, dentistry,

11

mirrors or photography.

As we move into the 21st century, Silver is finding many uses beyond those, but it is in the field of using colloids of Silver as a vital necessity to health, that we will explore further.

Survivors of the Black Death

Bubonic Plague has decimated world populations many times, but a peculiar fact about those terrible episodes was that royalty and heads of state had a far better survival rate than the peasantry, especially those who ate from Silver dishes or used Silver cutlery.

It was only in the late 18th century, when people began looking for something to kill bacteria that the reason for this better survival rate of royalty became clearer. Researchers discovered that Silver was the best thing they had ever found to kill every type of bacteria, fungi, or virus.

They then theorised that every time people ate acid foods such as stewed fruits stored in Silver dishes, the acids in the foods would dissolve some Silver from the utensil and these particles of Silver would be consumed with the meal.

Although this Silver was by no means colloidal, they were not ingesting enough to poison themselves. But they were taking in enough to kill many nasty pathogens, even though it was in large particle size compared to a colloid.

Argyria

A side effect of this Silver intake when excessive was a condition called Argyria. This is caused when Silver particles lodge under the skin, usually the fingernails and under the eyes, giving the skin a porcelain blue-grey colour.

This condition was with them for life, as there was no cure, nor does there appear to be an adequate one today. This peculiar skin colour is said to have given rise to the description of royalty as blue-bloods.

A modern case of Argyria

An American politician, Stan Jones developed a case of Argyria which received considerable media attention. It turned out he had been drinking four to six glasses of high ppm Colloidal Silver (made from tap water) every day for five years.

That's about 600 times the recommended amount of Silver entering his body.

He first noticed a blueness under his fingernails, and then a slight bluish tinge under his eyes and around his nose.

The skin colour was barely noticeable on his face. He complained that the media had digitally enhanced published pictures of him to bring out the blueness.

However the experiment in 1985 mentioned earlier, which involved drinking a litre a day of high ppm Colloidal Silver (made with distilled water) for weeks at a time, failed to produce any trace of Argyria in the original experimenter, nor in the other laboratory assistants who later repeated the experiment with the same results.

Only distilled water should be used to make Colloidal Silver for daily use. Using tap water produces an inferior product and should only be used for purification purposes. The Silver tends to form in large clumped particles which can be difficult for the body to eliminate, and blue-grey compounds such as Silver Chloride are often formed.

Industrial water purification

Silver electrodes are used in some Boeing commercial aircraft water purifying systems. Contaminated water is passed over an array of Silver electrodes to purify it.

This technique is also now being used overseas to purify swimming pool water. The result is bacteria–free water without any of the harm and stinging eyes of Chlorine.

A dramatic experiment along these lines was recently demonstrated in Nebraska – 250 litres of raw sewage water was pumped into a pool. The bacteria count (E-Coli) was measured at a high 7000 per 100 ml.

The sewage water was then flushed through an array of Silver electrodes. All bacteria were killed in less than 3 hours. Follow up tests showed that the water remained totally free of bacteria.

How does Colloidal Silver work?

Most people today have heard of food compounds called anti-oxidants or bioflavonoids. These are found in plants, especially fruits. Every moment of our lives cells split apart and give off atoms of oxygen in the process. These atoms of oxygen are eagerly sought after by cancer cells and other disease organisms which must have them to grow.

But they are also fiercely competed for by the anti-oxidants and bioflavonoids which depriving these pathogens of oxygen, slowing down their rate of growth.

Death by suffocation

Colloidal Silver has a similar effect, but works in a different manner. It would seem to have an everlasting hatred of all single celled pathogens, be they bacterial, fungal or viral. Silver too loves oxygen. The Silver colloids in the bloodstream seek out and surround their victims, smother them, and being totally deprived of all sustenance they suffocate and die.

Technical explanation of how it works

Here is a more technical explanation, taken from the Internet, as to how Colloidal Silver restores health in the cells of the body by killing disease organisms and viruses:

"In order to understand how Colloidal Silver works, one must first understand the disease state of the body. The body encounters pathogens and other foreign entities many times a day. When the body is healthy it maintains a proper pH and oxygen-rich environment."

"The pH (potential of Hydrogen) inside the cells of the body are usually near an alkaline 7.3. Outside the cell, the fluid surrounding the cells will usually realise an acidic pH, near 4.0."

"However, when an individual does not maintain a healthy environment in the body, the pH begins to rise in the outer fluid and fall inside the cell. This reduces the electrical potential of the cell."

"Oxygen levels in the cells respond by decreasing.

Pathogens (living disease organisms) that grow in the body will usually attack these weakened cells and 'set up shop'. These organisms, that cause illness and attack these weak cells, cannot survive in healthy cells that have outer fluid pH below 4.0 and inner cellular fluid above pH 6.9."

"Silver maintains a positive charge, which when introduced to areas of infection disrupt the pathogens causing the illness. Interestingly, Colloidal Silver kills the organisms by inhibiting the enzyme that these pathogens utilise to survive in their anaerobic (airless) environment. This enzyme is the pathogen's 'chemical lung'. Without the necessary enzyme for metabolism, growth, regeneration and survival, the pathogen 'suffocates' and dies."

"Viruses on the other hand, are destroyed, it is believed, because the electric charge of Silver particles causes their protective protein coat, also referred to as the 'head', to collapse. They are therefore unable to replicate, and are removed from the body by the immune, lymphatic, and intestinal elimination systems."

"This process is so effective that no pathogen has been recorded to mutate against Colloidal Silver, or live in its presence for more than six minutes. While antibiotics are losing their effectiveness as strains of germs become resistant to conventional antibiotics, they are not able to develop any resistant strains or immunity to Silver."

Resistance to antibiotics

Antibiotics work selectively on a few pathogens by poisoning them. In the course of this action they also kill off many useful body bacteria and enzymes. If the poison is not strong enough, and does not achieve a total kill, the surviving pathogens just shake their heads and refuse to indulge in the poison, or breed up a resistant strain and carry on with their evil designs.

There are many bacteria around now that laugh at almost every antibiotic that is fired at them. Also antibiotics in many cases, like most medical drugs often have nasty to severe side effects on the people to whom they are prescribed.

Can fungi, bacteria or viruses
build up resistance to Colloidal Silver?

No, not at all. Colloidal Silver has been with us now for over 100 years. All the tests have been done. There has never been a single case of any organism that could be killed by Colloidal Silver ever breeding resistance to it.

Why does the medical profession
keep using antibiotics?

The only reason I can think of, is that if they began using Colloidal Silver on a few patients, the good word would soon get around. Then other patients would demand it, and in a short time so many patients would be healed of their ailments that the doctors would suffer a drastic loss of income.

I suppose they keep solidly in mind a very true observation. *"A patient cured is a patient lost."*

It should also be kept in mind that Colloidal Silver is effective against viruses, yeasts or fungi, which antibiotics have never been. Nor do antibiotics speed up healing, as Colloidal Silver does.

If Colloidal Silver is so good
why do we need flu injections?

The day I discovered Colloidal Silver was the day I stopped getting flu injections.

We hear a lot of tripe about no cure for flu. Tell that to anyone who uses Colloidal Silver. In the three years or so I have been using Colloidal Silver I have never had so much as a sniffle.

What about the Super Bugs we are told about,
will Colloidal Silver kill them?

If it is a single cell pathogen, Colloidal Silver will kill it. As for the Super Bugs that we are told have killed over 100 patients in the last two years in our New Zealand hospitals, I do not believe any one of these people would have died had the medical profession known about and used Colloidal Silver.

Does Colloidal Silver help other bodily processes besides killing pathogens?

Yes, it would seem that Colloidal Silver is almost magical in assisting bodily health.

Doctor R.O. Becker, a highly respected biomedical researcher has written two books that I know of, **"The Body Electric"** and **"Cross Currents."** This is what he has written about his experiences with elderly patients, *"Colloidal Silver did more than kill disease-causing organisms. It promoted major growth of bone and accelerated the healing of injured tissues by over 50%."*

He also stated that Colloidal Silver, *"Profoundly stimulates healing in skin and other soft tissues in a way unlike any known natural process"* and that it *"promotes a new kind of cell growth that looks like the cells of children. These cells grew fast, producing a diverse and surprising assortment of primitive cell forms, able to multiply at a great rate, then differentiate into specific cells of an organ or tissue that had been injured, even in patients over 50 years old."*

Where antibiotics had proved useless

In a remarkable clinical trial with 14 elderly patients who had long-standing infections of bones to which antibiotics had proved useless, Dr R.O. Becker inserted two Silver electrode wires directly into each wound, using the body's own fluids as the liquid solution, and applied current to the external ends. The voltage used was so low it could not be felt. With this technique he was able to heal infections inside broken bones, one of the hardest type of infections to control. He was also able to mend previously non-healing fractures and breaks.

In some cases he left the Silver surgically implanted in the body. In others he sewed the wound up around the protruding electrode. Once the wound had healed, the Silver wire was pulled from the wound without any need for surgery or anaesthetics.

Regarding the ability of metallic Silver to heal infection he said, *"All the organisms we tested were sensitive to the electrically-generated Silver ions, including some that were*

17

resistant to all known antibiotics."

Concerning the safety of bodily insertion he said. *"In no case was any undesirable effects of the Silver treatment apparent."*

Do medical schools teach about colloids?

To the best of my knowledge, no. Almost all doctors, at least until recently, believed that Colloidal Silver was a poison, confusing it with the metal forms and compounds of the metal which are poisonous.

Medical compounds of Silver and other metals are sometimes added to external creams to try to kill bugs and viruses. Our bodies cannot break down these poisonous metal compounds, and if they are ingested they can accumulate in the body with dire consequences. A compound of Silver and a colloid of Silver are as different as chalk is from cheese.

Medical schools teach, correctly so, that Silver is a poison, but it is not a dangerous one. According to the New Zealand National Poison Centre it takes about 15 grams (½ oz) of Silver to poison an adult.

A by-product of Silver is used or generated in the photography industry and is called Silver Nitrate. This is much more poisonous. It reacts violently with body tissues and has a caustic effect. Just two grams can be fatal.

Colloidal Silver on the other hand is absorbed into the tissues with no irritation whatsoever.

How to make Colloidal Silver

Colloidal Silver is made by suspending 99.9% pure Silver rods (the highest purity available and known as Fine Silver) into 99.999997% pure distilled water. Water this pure should contain no more than 3 ppm (parts per million) of other minerals.

Tap water is usually contaminated with between 30 and 150 ppm of other minerals, even rainwater contains about 10 ppm of minerals.

When a low voltage electrical charge is placed across the rods, ions of Silver are drifted off in the process of electricity passing from one rod to the other. These 'ions' (that is why it is sometimes called 'ionic Silver') carry an electric charge and in that state the Silver remains suspended in the water.

Over a period of time, usually after three months, the Silver ions gradually lose their charge. For this reason Colloidal Silver is best used fresh.

Shaking before use is a good thing to practise with any liquid colloids, for when a Silver colloid is losing its electrical charge it can cling to the bottom or sides of the container. But even then, it is always better to use Colloidal Silver fresh. When it is carrying a full electrical charge it is absorbed much more quickly into the bloodstream.

Can colloids lose their charge in other ways?

Indeed they can. If Colloidal Silver is stored within the magnetic field of any large electrical device such as a TV, microwave, fridge or washing machine, the interference of the magnetic field can destroy the electrical charge on the Silver colloids.

How else can Colloidal Silver's effectiveness be destroyed?

Almost everyone has seen silverware gradually become blackened when exposed to air, particularly sulphurous air. Sulphur and Silver are attracted to one another and the end process is called oxidation. Because particles of Colloidal Silver are little more than atom size, particles of light (photons)

19

quickly oxidise Silver.

That is why it is absolutely essential to store Colloidal Silver in darkness, and preferably in a brown glass bottle. A good place to store it is in a drawer of clothing, or a closed cupboard.

In strong sunlight, a clear glass container of Colloidal Silver can be oxidised to uselessness in less than an hour. A gold solution will turn a purple grey or black. This is the same chemical process that makes black and white photography possible.

How can I make Colloidal Silver?

There are two methods of making Colloidal Silver. In both instances it is important to use 99.9% pure Silver rods.

A word of warning will not go astray here about the need to use pure Silver. Do not use jeweller's Sterling Silver, since it is only about 86% pure and contains copper and nickel. Nickel is poisonous and the ions coming from non-pure Silver rods may well be a much larger size, too big in fact to be called colloids.

A simple method of making Colloidal Silver

To make Colloidal Silver by a simple but crude method you will need to buy:

- Two pure Silver rods, about 4 to 6 inches long (approx 100 to 150 mm).
- Two lengths of insulated, electrical copper wire (with the capacity to carry a 9 volt direct current).
- A 9 volt battery (the kind used in smoke alarms which cost between $2 and $7).
- Two small crocodile clips.
- A Scotch Brite scouring pad from your supermarket. (Cut this into 2 inch squares with a sharp pair of scissors and use one of these pieces to clean your Silver rods after
  . using them to make Colloidal Silver.)

Strip the wires bare on each end to about half an inch and solder a Silver rod tip on one end, and a crocodile clip on the other end.

No, this is not a rough schoolboy hit and miss idea. This is how Dr R.C. Beck (not to be confused with Dr R.O. Becker) a scientist of impeccable credentials healed himself from serious illnesses by making Colloidal Silver and drinking what he made. Dr Beck claims that this is an ideal little portable Colloidal Silver generator you can take anywhere, especially if you are travelling overseas and water supplies are suspect. He claims you can even drink sewer water after treating it and have absolute confidence it is quite safe.

Sufficient to kill microbes

Next find a drinking glass or a small jar that has straight sides, or in other words as wide at the bottom as the top. Three quarters fill it with water straight from the tap, or if you are in the bush, straight from a stream or creek. Drop the Silver rods into the glass and position them about one inch (25 mm) apart and parallel to each other. Connect a crocodile clip to each terminal of the battery and you will be now making Colloidal Silver.

Set your watch for three minutes. By that time the water should have turned misty. Unclip your battery and remove the rods from the water. You now have a glass of Colloidal Silver.

Now this is not good quality Colloidal Silver. You need pure distilled water for that, but it is sufficient to kill microbes.

If at any time, using this method, the water turns grey or black, toss it away and try some other water. A mineral in the water has reacted with the Silver. It might be OK to use externally but do not drink it!

Pay special attention to this if you use this method

It is easy for this deceptively simple method to go wrong, and most people who make Colloidal Silver this way, with undistilled water are making an inferior product. Only use non-distilled water for emergencies or when you need to quickly purify suspect water.

This is because there are far too many mineral impurities in anything but distilled water. Most tap and stream water has between 30 and 150 ppm of elemental minerals such as Chloride, Calcium, Magnesium, Copper, etc.

Never add salt

Never add anything to the water that will increase its ability to conduct electricity. Not salt, not Celtic salt, not sea salt. Because salt puts Chloride ions in the water that react with the Silver to form Silver Chloride. Besides, because salt greatly speeds up the conductivity of electricity, it produces larger clumped particles, which are not true colloids. Therefore because of the presence of large particles, and the presence of Silver Chloride, it is best to avoid Silver products made with tap water or with added salt.

Which is more important, pure water or pure Silver?

Latest information is clear, it is water purity. Pure distilled water plays a larger part in producing pure Colloidal Silver than the purity of the Silver. So do not take any risks, use pure distilled water and 99.9% pure Silver, and use the preferred method of making Colloidal Silver whenever possible.

The preferred method of making Colloidal Silver

This second method is recommended by Dr R.C. Beck for making the best quality Colloidal Silver and is the method I use.

It takes longer than the crude method because pure distilled water does not contain minerals that greatly speed up the electrical conductivity of the water.

Purchase a professionally-made Colloidal Silver generator, a device about the size of a small transistor radio. These are not cheap, but it is a one off cost, and they are reliable, last for years, and are so convenient you can be making Colloidal Silver in your kitchen within a minute of receiving one.

The ones I use come from Sota Instruments in Canada, and as an agent I sell them to any person in New Zealand who may wish to acquire them. There are about 40 or 50 firms around the world who now make similar machines, I believe some are even made here in New Zealand.

The Canadian ones manufactured by Sota Instruments cost approximately $200 each.* Although Dr R.C. Beck invented

---

* This was the price of the Canadian units that Max was importing at the time. See page 78 for a high quality plug in mains generator couriered free.

22

these machines, he has no financial interest in any company who makes them. His sole interest is to get people using Colloidal Silver.

The machine comes fully operational, including the Silver rods, and batteries.

Before the Silver rods wear out they will make between 200 to 300 litres of Colloidal Silver. The batteries of course will need replacing as they wear out, but the heavy-duty grade batteries supplied usually last over a year in normal use. Replacement alkaline ones will last even longer.

Some units give you the option of also buying a little transformer that plugs into your mains electricity and bypasses the batteries. Useful if you are making large quantities.

Use only pure distilled water!

You will need to have a source of distilled water. You may have a distiller, or you can purchase 4 or 10 litre containers of distilled water from most supermarkets, or The Warehouse. Current prices are about 80c per litre for a ten litre container.

Pure Dew is a New Zealand brand of distilled water that has proven to be successful.

Be sure it is distilled water you buy and not mineral water. Otherwise the minerals in the water will combine with the highly reactive silver and you will not generate pure Colloidal Silver. More about this on the next page.

The only other thing you will need to find, or buy, is a glass jar. One that will hold between 500 mls and a litre (1000 mls) of distilled water. It also needs to be deep enough to allow for the length of the Silver rods on your machine. These are usually about five or six inches long (about 140 mm). An old Agee jam or preserving jar is ideal.

Now fill the jar with distilled water to about an inch from the top. This is important, because when the Silver rods are placed in the water they should have at least 75% of the rod immersed.

Should I heat the water?

The hotter the water the faster a given ppm of Colloidal Silver is generated. Simmering just below boiling point speeds up the process three times faster than at room temperature.

However unless you are making Colloidal Silver

23

commercially there is no point. It is a lot more trouble and there is a danger of scalding yourself, or damaging your generator.

Now to make your Colloidal Silver

Immerse the silver rods according to the instructions that came with your generator. They should be parallel to each other.

The rods should not touch the bottom or sides of the jar, as this encourages sediment to build up and flake off.

If the rods are too long they can be cut shorter, but always make sure they remain parallel to each other, i.e., the distance between the rods should remain about 1 to 1½ inches (24 to 38mm) along their full length.

At first the reaction proceeds very slowly. For 1 to 5 minutes nothing may seem to be happening. But you should soon see a smoke-like mist, drifting in the water around the positive silver rod.

If this mist appears in less than a minute, it is a sign that the water has too high a mineral content (over 2 ppm). You can proceed, but you will usually produce a greyish, unattractive Colloidal Silver that has combined negatively with other minerals in the water. It may still work as a germicide, but should not be taken internally, unless it becomes crystal clear, or has a transparent golden hue after standing overnight. Grey or brown Colloidal Silver has been found to be inferior in laboratory tests.

So provided it takes longer than a minute for the mist to appear, begin timing from this point.

Use the timer on your stove

It is easy to go away and forget that your generator is running. You may decide to use the timer and alarm on your stove as a reminder.

Why the mist can take a long time to appear

The mist normally appears within five minutes for recommended 2 ppm distilled water. But it can take very much longer for 1 ppm distilled water, or 0 ppm pharmaceutical grade ultra purified water. *

Water below 2 ppm barely conducts electricity, and you can wait for up to 2 to 4 hours as the machine struggles to build up enough silver to generate a workable current through the water. Before suspecting your generator of malfunctioning, do a test using tap water. Mist should quickly appear.

You can speed up the process and bring your distilled water up to 2 ppm of mineral content by adding about 5% filtered tap water. Or about 20% of previously made Colloidal Silver. This does not affect the quality of your Colloidal Silver.

Once the mist appears, the speed of generation is the same as that of 2 ppm distilled water.

Keep the rods clean

As well as the mist, some hydrogen bubbles may be seen coming from one of the silver rods (the one transmitting the positive current). The reaction will gradually speed up and the water will sometimes become cloudy.

While the silver rods are generating, the positive rod will accumulate a soft coating of dark grey oxide, and the other one a light brown coating. During the last third of the generating process the positive rod will become black and both rods should be taken out of the water and wiped with a paper towel or cloth. This prevents the black sediment from flaking off the positive rod and floating in the water. This wiping should ideally be done twice, or even three times.

The blackness is caused as oxygen particles in the water oxidise the Silver. If this is allowed to build up too much, (usually after 1 hour) it becomes thick enough dislodge from the rod and float in the water. It is easily filtered out however.

This accumulation on the rods does not appear to reduce their ability to generate Colloidal Silver.

How long do I leave the generator running?

Below are approximate guide times to use from the time the mist appears:

---

* Modern distilled waters are now 0 to 1 ppm and need filtered water added to bring them up to 2 ppm. The use of a PPM (parts per million) Meter is recommended for best results.

Container size	5 ppm	10 ppm
250 ml water	15 minutes	25 minutes
500 ml water	30 minutes	50 minutes
750 ml water	45 minutes	75 minutes
1 litre water	60 minutes	100 minutes
2 litres water	120 minutes	200 minutes

Using a ppm (parts per million) measuring meter

Some experimentation with generating time and water quality will probably be necessary until you gain experience. Or you can purchase a ppm Meter that measures the mineral content of the water and takes away the guesswork.

Nowadays you can buy battery-operated digital PPM Meters that accurately read the mineral content of water. These are high-tech instruments and are specially insulated against the ultra high conductivity of silver, so are not cheap. They cost almost as much as a Colloidal Silver generator, but they are simple to use and highly useful.

They look rather like an oversize pen. You just switch them on, dip the tip in the Colloidal Silver solution and it reads off the ppm in a little window like a digital watch. It takes all the guesswork out of making Colloidal Silver. *

A digital ppm Meter cannot tell you what the minerals are in the water, that requires a Spectrometer costing thousands of dollars. So to measure the ppm content of Silver in Colloidal Silver, you need to first measure the ppm content of the distilled water before you start generating the Colloidal Silver.

Distilled water typically measures between 1 to 2 ppm. Tap water by comparison usually measures between 30 ppm to over 100 ppm.

So to make 10 ppm strength Colloidal Silver from 2 ppm distilled water, you would run your Colloidal Silver generator until you obtain a reading of 12 ppm on the meter. In other words you subtract the starting ppm from the higher generated ppm.

Always stir the Colloidal Silver before taking a reading or you may get an artificially high reading.

---

* See page 79 for a top quality, well priced New Zealand made PPM Meter.

Filtering

When you have finished generating and have removed the rods, briefly stir the Colloidal Silver with a non-metal stirrer (the handle of a wooden spoon is ideal). Then filter out any black rod sediment from the solution by pouring it through a paper towel or clean cloth into another glass container. Or you can simply allow it to settle overnight and then pour off into a clean jar, leaving any sediment at the bottom.

Clean the Silver rods back to a shiny finish with a Scotch Brite pad before putting them away.

Guide to Colloidal Silver strength

Your Colloidal Silver may look cloudy at the end of the generating, but when it has been left to clear overnight, and any impurities have settled out, it should be clear and have a discernible golden hue when held up to the light and compared with plain water.

This will be more noticeable after 36 hours. Use this colour as your guide to strength. Just a hint of gold hue is all that is required for general use. This is normally a 5 ppm strength. A clear distinct gold colour is about 10 ppm. A deep gold is about 17 ppm.

If you ever leave the generator going too long and end up with a deep gold Colloidal Silver, you can dilute it back with additional distilled water. But do not dilute it more than 65% as there is natural limit of about 17 ppm when making Colloidal Silver from distilled water. After this limit is reached, the Silver just plates out onto the sides of the jar.

You will see this phenomena when using a ppm Meter. The ppm progresses steadily up to 17 ppm then is reluctant to go higher. The machine is still generating, but the Silver is plating out onto the glass walls of the jar, which can take on the appearance of a mirror.

Persistence for several hours more can push it over 20 ppm, but 17 seems to be a normal maximum, notwithstanding some overseas sales claims I have seen of 80 ppm. Colloidal Silver of this strength has certainly had other minerals, or a protein - like gelatine added to artificially boost the levels.

If you try generating the Colloidal Silver again the next day you can generally force it up to 24 ppm. This is good for a high-strength gel, but a 5 to 10 ppm concentration is sufficient to kill pathogens and is all you need for most purposes.

Making Colloidal Silver suitable for intravenous injections

For intravenous injections you should use double-distilled 0 ppm Pharmaceutically Pure water from a chemist (as mentioned above) to make your Colloidal Silver. You will probably need to wait patiently for about two hours until the light comes on before starting your timing.

How to store Colloidal Silver

Once you have made high quality Colloidal Silver you need to protect it so that the Silver particles maintain their positive electrical charge and remain separate from each other in suspension.

Like charges repel each other and anything that removes this positive charge from the particles such as ultraviolet light from the sun, magnetic fields of home appliances like refrigerators, and also some cheap plastics, will degrade the effectiveness of the Colloidal Silver by causing the particles to clump together and become too large to be fully effective. These things can also cause gold Colloidal Silver to darken to a grey or purple colour, especially the effects of sunlight.

Colloidal Silver is therefore best stored out of the fridge, in a dark glass container. Beer or ginger beer bottles are ideal.

Clear glass and high quality PET plastic can also be used, even the jar you use to generate it in, provided it is kept in a dark place such as a closed cupboard or drawer, or in a lightproof cardboard carton.

Before bottling, stir the Colloidal Silver with a wooden spoon, or plastic spatula to ensure that the colloids are well distributed. Never use metal as this can affect the electric charge.

Is it possible to manufacture different sizes of Silver colloids?

Some people make sales claims that their colloids are a smaller size than what others can make. Any science book I have ever read states that when a low voltage electric charge is applied to pure Silver rods in water, the size of the particles drifting off never varies. It will always be .001 microns. (Voltage during generating should not exceed 35 volts.)

It is the clumping together of colloids that causes large particles. That is why it is essential to use pure Silver and extremely pure water.

Also store Colloidal Silver away from sunlight and magnetic fields, and ideally use it within three months for maximum benefit.

How expensive is Colloidal Silver to make?

Well lets work it out. Presume you buy a generator and decide to use the distilled water method.

A Silver generator costs about $200* and usually makes a litre (1000mls) of Colloidal Silver in about two hours.

Let's say you buy your distilled water from the supermarkets. Say $4 for four litres. The Silver rods will make between 200 and 350 litres, probably nearer 350 than 200 before replacements are needed. Replacement rods cost about $20.

So let's work out our price to make 200 litres of Colloidal Silver. That's 200,000 mls or 40,000 teaspoons and should last one person over 50 years at two teaspoons a day.

Let us also say we toss the Silver generator away after making 200 litres, although in fact it would probably turn out at least another 400 litres before some small replacement was needed.

Water $200
Generator $200
Batteries $45
Total cost $445
Amount manufactured =200 litres (200,000 mls).
Cost per litre $2.23

Think about it. If you were using a 300 ml bottle of bought Colloidal Silver a month, at $20 to $50 a bottle ($67 to $167 a litre) it would be a sound, money-saving investment to outlay the money to make your own.

---

* This was the price of a Canadian unit that Max was importing at the time. See page 78 for a quality New Zealand made generator couriered free.

How do I make gold Colloidal Silver?

Provided you use pure distilled water and pure silver rods there is no reason why your Colloidal Silver will not turn out gold if you generate it above 5 ppm.

Increasing your generating time by 25% should give you about 10 ppm which normally produces a beautiful gold colour. You need to allow 36 hours for the full colour to develop.

10 ppm Colloidal Silver has a slightly metallic taste.

Why are Silver colloids gold?

It has long been considered a mystery why Colloidal Silver turns gold at higher concentrations.

It is also a mystery why any colour at all is seen when there are only five parts of silver in a million. For example, if you stood on a bridge and looked down into a river where there was a school of a million transparent fish, stretching from bank to bank and as far up the river as the eye could see, and there were only five gold fish included among the school, (that's one gold fish to every 200,000 transparent fish). You would hardly expect to see the five gold ones among the hundreds of thousands of transparent ones, even if all the other fish were invisible. However, perhaps if we are comparing millions to trillions in a confined space we will see some colour.

Several theories have been suggested to explain the gold appearance of Colloidal Silver. Some claim the Silver particles are too large, due to clumping. But this appears highly unlikely. That would reduce our five goldfish to just one or two large ones, even less visible.

Others say it is contamination from other minerals in the water. But even using 0 ppm ultra-pure water, the gold colour still appears.

Some suggest that it is contaminating sulphur from the Silver rods. But this cannot be true either, for the gold is obviously Silver, because it turns blue-black in sunlight, just as Silver does in black and white photography.

Yellow a sign of the optimum range of colloid effectiveness

A 1926 English book entitled *"Practical Colloid*

Chemistry" under the section **'Polychromism of Silver Solutions'** states *"the continuous change in colour from yellow to blue, corresponds to a change in the absorption maximum of the shorter to longer wave lengths, with a decreasing degree of dispersion."*

It then goes on to say that the particle size range that can appear yellow is .001 up to .01 microns, as those sizes absorb indigo light, leaving only its inverse colour yellow to be observed. The yellow appears only when the particles have been evenly dispersed.

This explanation makes sense, for when exposed to sunlight, yellow Colloidal Silver turns blue-black. A reliable sign that the particles have clumped together into much larger particles, which now reflect the blue end of the spectrum.

The yellow-gold size range of particles, .001 up to .01 size is the optimum range of effectiveness. Professor R. J. Gibbs, director of The Center for Colloidal Science, University of Delaware who has published over 85 peer-reviewed journal articles on colloidal minerals states, *"The ideal Colloidal Silver product would be made up of particles less than .01 micron, and preferably ranging from .01 to .001. The product should be in distilled water with no additional dissolved substances other than the Silver particles."*

What is the correct dosage?

Well, there is no such thing as maximum or minimum doses; it depends on size. An average size adult who had never used it before, and had not been using other colloidal minerals would for a certainty be very short of it in their body.

So if you have never used Colloidal Silver before I would suggest you start with one teaspoon a day (5ml), and double that dose daily until you are taking ten teaspoons a day (50ml), which would be gladly welcomed by your body. Then continue to take ten teaspoons a day for a week. From then on, purely from a maintenance point of view, two teaspoons (10ml) a day should suffice.

But if you were working in an office where a nasty flu was doing the rounds, I would take ten teaspoons a day.

I would also carry my little spray bottle with me, and at the first sign of a sniffle or tickle in the throat, I would pump a few puffs up each nostril, then open my mouth and while breathing in slowly, spray a generous amount onto my tonsils. (See page 37 regarding the use of an empty Beconase spray bottle, or other spray bottle.)

Dosages

In 1940, R.A. Kehoe reported that in normal circumstances the average daily intake of fruits and vegetables would provide between 50-100 micrograms of Colloidal Silver as a trace element.

Since that time commercial farm soils in almost all nations have become very to extremely deficient in trace minerals. According to Earth Summit report in 1992, the levels of soil-based minerals in the older settled eastern areas of the USA have dropped 85% in the last 100 years.

Assuming earlier generations had a more adequate diet of trace minerals than we obtain from our foods today, there is sound argument to supplement with Colloidal Silver, and other trace minerals too for that matter.

Two teaspoons a day

Two teaspoons of 5 ppm Colloidal Silver works out at about

50 mcg of Colloidal Silver, and this could be a nutritional amount if taken daily. Most household teaspoons are smaller than the true metric teaspoon which holds 5 mls.

Two metric teaspoons equal one dessertspoon (10 mls) and three teaspoons equal one tablespoon (15 mls). Most dessertspoons are reasonably accurate as a measure of two metric teaspoons. (Use a plastic teaspoon where possible.)

Any amount above four teaspoons daily should be regarded as a therapeutic amount.

If you wish to experiment with larger amounts, do so with caution. I take over 150 mls (ten tablespoons a day) and have experimented with that for a year with only beneficial effects, but what suits one may not help another.

If you have to buy your Colloidal Silver, I always say one teaspoon a day until a virus or bacteria attempts to attack, and then saturate yourself with it for a few days.

If you are making it yourself you can afford to be more generous and take two teaspoons a day.

Effectiveness

Colloidal Silver's effectiveness is directly related to the size of the particles. 10 million colloids of Silver size .001 microns can fit into the space taken by a Silver particle size of 1 micron. Thus the smaller the particle size, the better the coverage for destroying pathogens.

Particle size, plus the stability of the positive charge of electricity on the Silver ions decide just how effective your Colloidal Silver will be.

Also as mentioned earlier, it is very important to keep your Colloidal Silver away from sunlight and all electrical and magnetic interference. TV's, microwaves, stoves and fridges are very bad companions for Colloidal Silver as their magnetic fields can cause your Silver particles to clump together.

Digestive interaction

Millions of people take Colloidal Silver on a daily basis with no sign of stomach upset, even after prolonged use.

I have however read of two persons who took one teaspoon and complained of tummy upset, but this is very rare.

There are two ways to avoid the possibility of tummy upset if you have a sensitive stomach. The first way is to swish the Colloidal Silver around in your mouth for about a minute and a half. This helps the Silver colloids to move into your bloodstream directly from under your tongue, thus by-passing the stomach.

The other way is to take multiple small doses a day.

Will Colloidal Silver kill friendly bacteria?

Many people think that Colloidal Silver will kill friendly bacteria in the stomach. But our body's friendly bacteria are found in our intestines rather than the stomach. The stomach is a hostile place for bacteria due to powerful digestive acids. In fact research has shown that Colloidal Silver being ionised, is absorbed before it enters the small intestine, unless we drink huge amounts.

Yes in theory Colloidal Silver will kill friendly bacteria, but in reality it does not happen. Even when high dosages are taken. If it did happen, a plate of Acidophilus yoghurt would soon get things right.

How can I get Colloidal Silver into my intestines?

A number of diseases such as cholera, canine parvovirus where the pathogen resides mainly in the intestines are fatal, mostly due to the dehydration resulting from prolonged diarrhoea and or vomiting.

The pathogen causing the problem is active in the large intestine, the one place where Colloidal Silver when used as normally recommended, will NOT penetrate.

You can get Colloidal Silver into the intestines by drinking a one off dose of 200 ml (a full tea cup) of Colloidal Silver added to 500ml of water, on an empty stomach first thing in the morning, then immediately lying down for twenty minutes. This should give almost immediate relief from the worst symptoms. Then consume half a litre of Acidophilus yoghurt.

How much would I give a month old baby with the flu?

Remember it is not a poison, but if it was my baby I would use a fine mist sprayer and spray three or more puffs into its mouth each half hour or so. The baby would swallow a little of it and a trace may be breathed into the lungs which could only do good.

Are there any side effects from Colloidal Silver?

While I personally have never seen any, I have read that if a person has severe symptoms of an illness and they take a large dose of Colloidal Silver, what is called a 'Healing Crisis' can occur. This is when the person experiences flu-like symptoms; headache, extreme fatigue, dizziness, aching muscles and nausea.

This is because Colloidal Silver is attacking all the foreign enemies in your body at once. If you have an excess of enemies in your blood killed off too soon because you have taken a large dose of Colloidal Silver, traffic jams may occur in your cleansing system. Our body eliminates toxins, poisons and wastes through the liver, kidneys, lungs, skin and bowels.

You might be surprised to know that the average person's body is loaded with about half a pound of 'aliens'. They can be tape worms, liver fluke, bowel worms, Hepatitis C, E Coli., Typhoid, Streptococci, Lupus, etc.

So if as a first time user you develop some of these symptoms, increase your distilled water intake to ensure bowel movement, reduce your intake of sugar and unnatural fats like margarine, and reduce your Colloidal Silver intake to a teaspoon a day until the symptoms clear.

Have you ever seen failures with Colloidal Silver?

Yes, a person had Scabies. We didn't know what it was. It looked like some sort of rash and was itchy. They dabbed some Colloidal Silver on and got relief, and took a teaspoon, morning and night. It didn't work. Why?

Well firstly, they had never taken Colloidal Silver before in their lives. Their body at the age of 78 would be chronically short of it. They had as it turned out, Scabies all over their body. They would have needed to drink at least two half glasses a day to combat the constant re-infection.

They would also have needed to sterilise all clothing and blankets etc, to prevent constant re-infection, and to have sprayed all furniture and carpets with Colloidal Silver to kill the bugs in the house. But I believe that had their body like mine, been saturated with the Silver colloid, they would never have caught it.

Another man aged 82 had Psoriasis all over his body. He only showed me his arms and I could see his head was totally covered in it too. We rubbed his arms with Colloidal Silver and sprayed his head and eyes and he expressed great relief. The next I heard he was in hospital.

Again, with a body that had never had access to Silver in his life, he would have needed to drink four glasses a day to combat such an infection.

I have had five or six other people who have told me they have used Colloidal Silver and it had not helped at all.

Doctor Gary Smith, a Colloidal Silver research pioneer has noticed a very definite correlation between low levels of Silver in the body and an inability to ward off illness. Dr Smith who uses Colloidal Silver to treat his cancer patients says, *"Success depends on the amount of Silver in a person's body, and failures result from a lack of Silver in the body."*

Have you ever heard of people resistant to Colloidal Silver?

I have read where, on a rare occasion a person will be found to whom the colloid does not agree with. On two occasions I have heard that when it was sprayed in the eyes they became inflamed.

Note however, that no person has ever died from using Colloidal Silver, nor did these two people. But it is pointless using any substance if it causes swelling or inflammation. I would say to such people, "Do not use it."

I tell people to put some in their eyes with a dropper, or to spray some in. It should not sting at all. If it should sting for any longer than a second, then don't use it!

What is the quickest way to get Colloidal Silver where it's needed?

The best place to have Colloidal Silver is in your blood. The quickest way to get it there is through an injection into the blood. This would need to be done by a doctor. I doubt if any doctor has done it, or would do it, so you have to forget that method.

The next quickest way to get anything into your blood is by holding it under your tongue. You can do this by taking about half a mouthful and holding it under your tongue for a minute or so, swallow it and repeat the dose.

However Colloidal Silver will eventually find its way into your blood when swallowed.

A useful little spray bottle you can carry around with you

If you have hay fever, sinus trouble, a sore throat, or a heavy dose of the flu, a most valuable aid is a spray bottle you can carry around with you. The best bottle I have discovered for this purpose is an empty 'Beconase' spray bottle.

'Beconase' is a drug doctors sometimes prescribe for Asthmatics or people with hay fever or sinus troubles. It is in a small glass brown bottle about two inches (50mm) in height with a plastic sprayer which puts out an extremely fine spray.

If you cannot obtain one from someone who uses them and tosses them away, then go to a chemist and buy one. Pour the drug down the drain because you only want the sprayer. That means it will cost you about $22 for an empty bottle, but it will be worth every cent. * (See footnote below for cheaper option.)

Breath spray into your nose and throat and your cold symptoms will vanish

After you have thoroughly soaked and washed the bottle and the plastic sprayer in hot water, you will have a handy glass bottle you can carry in handbag or pocket.

Fill it with Colloidal Silver and at the first sign of a cold, sore throat, or hay fever, spray several pumps in the air in front of your face and breath the fine vapour into your lungs, first through your nose and then through your mouth.

Do this every hour, or as often as you like and your symptoms will vanish like snow in the desert.

---

* Health House, suppliers of the Colloidal Silver generator and PPM meter (see pages 78 and 79, can supply Colloidal Silver in small, reusable, blue, glass-equivalent PET plastic spray bottles.

The sprayer is also excellent to spray into your eyes at any sign of infection, or if they feel tired, or if you are driving for any length of time. It refreshes them.

Colloidal Silver used in a nebuliser to treat Asthma and Pneumonia

Colloidal Silver is now being used overseas in nebulisers to help those who suffer from asthma.

Dr Marcial-Vega reports that he has used Colloidal Silver nebuliser treatments on infants, the elderly, and patients with pneumonia and has seen great results. All have responded quickly to the treatment even when no other approach seemed to help.

No one has reported any adverse reactions. He says that two 15 minute sessions per day will normally produce positive results from the very first day.

Testimonials of disorders cured or greatly eased by Colloidal Silver

The proverb *"Those who cannot remember the lessons of history are doomed to repeat them"* never holds so true as in the field of medicine. Do people like me have to note and record all the things that have been relieved or healed by the use of the Colloidal Silver?

Where are all the medical records of the early 1900's? Why should private citizens have to teach doctors what they should be taught in medical school? All the research has been done and I am quoting from old history when I quote these figures.

Over 650 problems can be successfully dealt with by use of Colloidal Silver. I have not the slightest doubt that were more testing to be done today, many more could be added to the list. Here are just a few documented in Medical Journals. 183 references compiled by Dr A.B. Flick MD can be found on the internet at www.svpvril.com/AgBIBLIO.html.

Acne
Aids
Allergies
Appendicitis
Arthritis rheumatoid
Asthma
Athletes foot
Bad breath
Bed sores
Bladder infection
Blood parasites
Blood poisoning
Boils
Bone cancer
Bowel disorders
Breast Cancer
Bubonic plague
Burns
Cancer

Candida
Chilblains
Cholera
Chronic Fatigue
Colitis
Conjunctivitis
Contact lens infections
Cuticle Infection
Cuts and wounds
Cystitis
Dandruff
Dermatitis
Diabetes
Diphtheria
Dysbiosis
Dysentery
Ear infections
Eczema
Emphysema

Epstein Barr virus
Encephalitis
Epiditymitis
Erysipelas
Eye infections
Fibrositis
Foot odour
Furunculosis
Gastritis
Glaucoma
Glue ear
Gonorrhea
Gum disease
Hay fever
Haemorrhoids
Herpes
Hives
Impetigo
Indigestion
Influenza
Intestinal disorders
Irritable bowel syndrome
Keratitis
Keratosis
Leg ulcers
Leprosy
Leukaemia
Lupus
Lyme disease
Lymphangitis
Malaria
Mastitis
ME
Measles
Meniers symptoms
Meningitis
Mouth ulcers
Mumps
Nappy rash
Neurasthenia
Nose infections

Ophthalmia (purulent)
Paget's disease
Parasite infections
Parvovirus (canine)
Pink Eye
Pleurisy
Pneumonia
Prostate enlarged
Psoriasis
Quinsy
Respiratory Infections
Rheumatism
Rhinitis
Ringworm
Scarlet fever
Scarletina
Seborrhea
Sepsis
Septicaemia
Shingles
Skin cancer
Skin rashes
Sinus infections
Sores
Spruce
Staph infections
Stomach flu
Stomach ulcers
Strep infections
Streptococcus infections
Sunburn
Sunspots
Syphilis
Throat infections
Thrush
Thyroid infections
Tonsillitis
Tooth ache
Toxaemia
Trachoma
Traveller's diarrhoea

Trench foot
Tuberculosis
Typhoid
Urinary infections
Ulcers
Under arm odour

Vaginal infections
Viruses (all forms)
Warts
Whooping cough
Yeast infections

Have you personal evidence of the efficacy of Colloidal Silver?

Yes. Some two years ago I had Conjunctivitis that used to laugh at antibiotics. A friend sprayed some Colloidal Silver in my eyes three times in half an hour and the eyes became brand new. Just magic!

Have you had letters from users?

Yes. Consider these. I have no permission to print names but these are extracts from letters I have received.

Sinus and Cystitis

"I gave some Colloidal Silver to a friend of mine and she rang me a couple of days later to tell me that a terrible type of Catarrh-type Sinus had vanished! Colloidal Silver can perform miracles. My Cystitis has again been cured by Colloidal Silver." BE

Glaucoma

"I thought you would like to know that I saw the eye specialist last week and she was surprised at the results of the tests. When I saw her six months ago the pressure in my right eye was 24. This time it was 18. The pressure in my left eye was 18, now it is 14. I shall continue to bathe them in the eye bath twice a day with Colloidal Silver. Sincere thanks for the help you have given me."

MV

Dental root canal filling

"Recently I had a dental X-ray, and was told I would have to have a root canal filling. I quickly took to the Colloidal Silver, and the dentist was very surprised when he noticed the abscess receding. He asked me if I was on antibiotics. I said, 'No."

"I almost died laughing when I saw his face. It was just one huge question mark written all over his face! He couldn't fathom

41

it out. Thank you for everything." CMH

Shingles

I received a phone call from an 86 year old woman asking if I could do anything to help her with her Shingles. I told her I was not a doctor, just a well-read retired farmer. She expressed gratitude that I was not a doctor because she said she had spent hundreds of dollars on doctors for a nil result. She told me she had Shingles in both breasts and on the back of her shoulder. She had not slept for one year except for brief periods before the pain woke her again. She was desperate and asked could I suggest anything at all. I told her I believed Colloidal Silver would help her. I sent her some Colloidal Silver with instructions to take three teaspoons a day and gradually increase the dose. She took three tablespoons the day she received it.

I received a phone call next day to say she had gone to bed and slept for eight hours. She has continued to take the Colloidal Silver at a maintenance rate of a teaspoon a day.

I received a letter from her some months ago. She had regained the two and a half stone she had lost over her Shingles ordeal, and is playing golf again. She says the Shingles has not totally vanished, she still gets a faint twitch now and then, but after the pain she had been through it is easily bearable.

Sore eyes

"I have tried the Silver and I feel like a new woman, which is true. Also I put it in my eyes as they were very sore and it fixed them immediately." BE

Lupus

"My wife has suffered the pains of hell for 15 years. She has had to endure all sorts of tests, and experiment with innumerable drugs. No matter what they threw at her it didn't cure. It alleviated, and with side effects I might add, but if she didn't take it, back it would come."

"What sort of people have we training doctors and running our medical schools that an old retired farmer like you can give her something that turns her into a new woman? How come you know about Colloidal Silver and they don't? She has thrown away her drugs, only takes Colloidal Silver now, and no side effects. Thanks a million." HA

Paget's disease

"Thank you so much for sending that Colloidal Silver for Mushke (her dog). *She is completely cured now, and no brown marks on her pretty little face.* (The dog had continually weeping eyes that nothing offered by the vets could heal)."

"So much for the dog, I have got Paget's disease of the bones, and I broke my leg in June and I have had quite a lot of pain for years with this condition as I lead a very busy life. Never enough hours in the day."

"Well I took some of your Colloidal Silver and found I could get out of a chair, or garden without pain. It seems silly, but I tried to remember when I was without pain; just part of your life. So how can I thank you for what you have done."

"I am going to tell my vets about this." GP

Testimonials from doctors

A Kansas doctor

"We have had instant success with Colloidal Silver and immune- compromised patients. A few examples are: Pink Eye; totally resolved in less than six hours (topical)."

"Recurrent Sinus Infections; resolved in eight days (oral ingestion)."

"Acute Cuticle Infection; resolved in 24 hrs (topical)."

"Another major area in which we have improved our clinical results is in the area of bowel detoxification and Dysbiosis."

"The Colloidal Silver has proved excellent for the removal of abnormal Intestinal Bacteria."

"Also it has proved to a great adjunct to our Candida Albicans, Epstein Barr virus, and Chronic Fatigue syndrome protocols."

Dr Gary Fischback MD

"I have had occasion to use this compound in my practice. I have used it to treat viral Pharyngitis (sore throat), infections of the ear canal, sinus infections, conjunctivitis (eye infection) and topically for skin infections. In virtually every case resolution was swift and complete. And while many antibiotics have profound side effects, Colloidal Silver has none."

Dr. Richard L. Davies, director Utah Silver Institute.

"In four years we have described 87 important new medical uses for silver. We are just beginning to see to what extent silver can relieve suffering and save lives."

Dr Albert Cullum MD.
"In every instance in which Colloidal Silver has been used by me, it has been successful. Even when antibiotics failed."

Dr Harry Markgraf MD
"Silver is the best germ fighter we have."

Testimonials from elsewhere

Contact lens infections
"After years of adverse reactions to contact lenses and having eye infections which prescriptions didn't solve, my eyes are now snowy white."

Eye infection in dogs
"My two very old Yorkshire Terriers have had sore eyes for 3½ years. I have been to several different vets including an eye specialist for animals and used dozens of little tubes of eye ointments with no results from any of them. Since I have used Colloidal Silver they have cleared up with no more pus. Unbelievable after all the stuff I've put in them before."

Colds, Flu, Allergies and Asthma
"We all take our daily dose, including our daughters aged eight and four, We have not had any colds or flu since taking the Silver eight months ago, and my husband has not had his allergies this season. My eight year old has not used her inhaler for months now! We feel great and want to share this discovery."

Psoriasis
"The Psoriasis has faded. I don't seem to be so tired either."

Warts
"My daughter's two biggest Warts have gone. I personally have been feeling much healthier overall."

Eczema

"My son Scotty has had badly inflamed Eczema around his mouth but the Silver cleared it up right away."

A woman had suffered from eczema for years. She had tried many remedies but without success. One day a friend told her about Colloidal Silver for eczema. She tried it and it worked! She found that the itching and desire to scratch disappeared immediately, and soon the dryness was gone and the sore red blotches turned a healthy pink.

"I had an area of Varicose Eczema on my left leg and that has cleared up as well. I would have no hesitation in recommending Colloidal Silver to anyone, no matter what the complaint may be." JH

Eczema in animals

"I am a dog lover and thought, if Colloidal Silver is good enough for me, it's good enough for my dogs. So I put some Colloidal Silver in my dog's water bowls as well. I have two small dogs. One of my dogs suffers from eczema and scratches constantly. I also sprayed it on his coat and rubbed it in."

"I noticed within a day or so, no more scratching and the redness to his skin is gone and better still – no more bad doggy breath. I have also noticed they both seem to have more energy, so thanks. woof woof!!" TA

Sun spots

"The Sun Blemish on the back of my hand has cleared so dramatically that it is less than a quarter of its size before I began putting Colloidal Silver on it each day. Great stuff eh?"

"My Spine and other moving parts of my body are so much more mobile and less painful. I thank God he directed me to you and your Colloidal Silver."

Asthma

"A minute ago I used the peak flow meter to measure my lung function and obtained a reading of 330 l/m, already a major improvement from the 250 l/m, and after just two weeks of Colloidal Silver."

Bladder Cancer

"Two years ago I was diagnosed with Bladder Cancer. I had an ultra sound which exposed a 42mm diameter tumour in my

bladder. It was suggested that my bladder be removed and I would therefore be left with an external bladder bag. This was most distressing for me."

"In the three weeks leading up to my operation I consumed 100ml (about 7 tablespoons) of Colloidal Silver per day (yes I was over-doing it, but I was in panic mode). Then came time for the operation and I was prepared for the worst."

"Before the operation, they performed a camera search inside my bladder. This search revealed that the tumour had reduced significantly in size. The surgeon said to me, "Whatever you have been doing, continue doing it." Then he said, "That is truly a miracle.""

"Today, two years later, I have just had another camera scan and I am still free of Cancer. Again the surgeon said, "Keep on doing what you're doing and I'll see you next year.""

"I consume daily for good health 30ml (2 tablespoons) and I thoroughly recommend Colloidal Silver." SB Australia

Bad Breath

After four days of taking Colloidal Silver a user realised his mouth tasted sweeter, whereas he usually had a bad taste in his mouth. His breath was sweeter, actually pleasant. The only thing different he had done was to begin taking Colloidal Silver daily.

About a week after his bottle was empty, the sour taste returned to his mouth and the bad breath came back. He quickly remedied that by getting back onto his daily regimen of Colloidal Silver.

Bone and Liver cancer

"My wife has been undergoing chemotherapy for Cancer. She was constantly tired and nauseous. At one stage she was unable to have her fortnightly chemotherapy due to a low white blood cell count. After checking with her physician, we were given the go ahead for her to try Colloidal Silver. She started with a tablespoon of Silver every morning. Her nausea vanished and she was able to begin her chemotherapy again."

"There was Cancer in the liver and bone, after two weeks she had blood tests and subsequent results revealed that her liver condition had improved by 50%, and the bone condition had improved by 30%. We hope that this information will be of

46

assistance in bringing this amazing product to the general public."

KW

Hair Re-growth during Chemotherapy

"I have Cancer and am receiving conventional treatment by chemotherapy. My hair began falling out as a side effect of this treatment. One month after taking Colloidal Silver on a daily basis, I realised my hair was growing back, and now I have once again a full head of hair. Other effects of the chemotherapy such as weight gain and fluid retention also seem to be of a much lesser degree with the Colloidal Silver." NC

Candida

"I suffered from Candida Albicans for a year before it was diagnosed and my symptoms were many and various. They varied from spots in front of my eyes, to bloating and fatigue to name just a few."

"I work in a health food store and was constantly looking for ways to self treat, because what I was prescribed was just not working. I had seen the Colloidal Silver on the shelf and after reading that Silver is an anti-fungal, anti-viral and anti-bacterial I decided that I had nothing to lose by trying it."

"I was taking only one teaspoon in a bottle of water and not making a lot of progress. So I increased the dose to 10ml three times daily for four days, then again stepped up to 20mls (4 teaspoons) three times daily for the next three months. I also avoided all sugars, fruit, dairy, alcohol, caffeine and gluten. I supplemented it with acidophilus capsules."

"On my last visit to my practitioner I was told that the yeast overgrowth in my system had gone and that Candida was no longer a problem. I am convinced that if I had not taken the Colloidal Silver, I would still be fighting the Candida." Cath

Skin Cancer

"I gave one bottle (of Colloidal Silver) to a New Zealand friend living in Bali. It has helped clear up a little Skin Cancer she had operated on and which appeared to be growing again." JM

Diabetes

A 68 year old woman had suffered with Diabetes for 25

years. She used insulin, both tablet and injection. Although she was careful with her diet, she was bedridden most of the time due to her Diabetes. Her husband began giving her a teaspoon of Colloidal Silver daily. With no other change in her lifestyle she soon felt more vigorous and began getting out of bed and being active during the day. Then she began to have insulin reactions, like those she would have if she administered too much insulin. So she cut back on the amount of insulin and continued her daily Colloidal Silver. The insulin reactions continued and she again reduced her insulin intake. Finally when her insulin doses had dropped to about a fourth of what they had been, the reactions stopped, and she has taken the lesser amount ever since.

Talking with other Diabetics, she found the younger Diabetics with less severe conditions who also were taking daily Colloidal Silver had ceased taking insulin altogether. Their conditions remained improved when they took no insulin, but only as long as they continued taking their Colloidal Silver regimen.

Ear infection

"I developed a particularly nasty infection in my ear. At first it was just sore, then it swelled up and hearing became difficult. Finally I experienced pain all over the left side of my face."

"During the following week I visited the doctor three times, receiving two types of ear drops and a course of antibiotics as treatment. After completing the prescribed course, the swelling and tenderness was still there."

"A friend of my mother's recommended Colloidal Silver, sprayed directly into the ear. After three days of spraying, three times a day (and placing a cotton ball soaked in Colloidal Silver in there as well) the swelling and pain disappeared completely. I had not used any other medication during those three days."

"Now I don't know if it's coincidence or not, but it worked and I will continue to use it for general health." DC

Emphysema

"I drink Silver every day, and am now using it in my jet nebuliser, taking the vapours directly into my lungs. I have a rare form of genetic Emphysema that is quite severe. My doctors and nurses shake their heads when they listen to my lungs and hear

48

how well they are working! Need I say more?" Darcy, Virginia, USA

"I have Emphysema. Over the past two years I have been hospitalised four times with chest infections, coughing and bringing up mucous. My sister sent me a book on Colloidal Silver. That was six months ago and I am happy to say that Colloidal Silver has definitely helped me. The coughing has stopped, the mucous has dried up, and life is a lot more pleasant." JH

Irritable Bowel Syndrome
"Over the past few years I have developed Irritable Bowel Syndrome. It is a month since I commenced taking Colloidal Silver. I have noticed much improvement as most of my nausea, stomach cramps and diarrhoea have gone." AVD

Old dog given up for dead
A vet had given a woman's old Schnauzer dog up for dead and sent her home to die. He said he could do no more for the dog. That was the day the woman first received Colloidal Silver and she decided to try some on her miserable pet. She gently fed a small amount of the Silver to the weakened animal. Within an hour the Schnauzer was showing signs of life. The sparkle returned to her eyes and in a very short time she was her old healthy self again, eating and fetching the stick.

Dog bites
"Our English setter was horribly attacked by a pack of Rottweiler's. Over 300 bites and one wound requiring 80 stitches. He developed a gangrenous type of infection in one of the bite sites and the vet had really given up all hope that the dog could survive the severity of the attack. I began infusing Colloidal Silver into the wounds, and giving him a couple of teaspoons to drink daily, and he recovered in no time."

Psoriasis, Warts and Sunspots
"Having been a Psoriasis sufferer for many years, I was resigned to the fact that I would probably always have it. Nothing I had used in the past had made much difference. However, after using Colloidal Silver, both internally and externally I was delighted to find that my Psoriasis patches were beginning to clear. After about three months they had all but disappeared."

"I have also had very good results with the application of

49

Colloidal Silver on warts and sunspots. " BA

Respiratory Infections (using a Nebuliser)
"Simply add 10ml (2 teaspoons) of Colloidal Silver into your nebulizer instead of your Ventolin or other prescription medication. Administer as you would normally and you should find yourself experiencing almost immediate results."

"We have received wonderful feedback from many sufferers who are now symptom free. If in doubt, talk to your doctor." Colloidal Silver manufacturer in Australia.

Sinus problems
"I have suffered from Sinus and Sinusitis for as long as I can remember, often taking Panadol on a daily basis to try and combat the effects of constant aching sinus and not being able to think clearly due to the congestion. "

"I have been worried for some time about the long term effects on my health of taking pain killers and antihistamines for prolonged periods and the effect they must be having on my kidneys and liver. "In my desperation I picked some Colloidal Silver up from my local health shop in Perth. I started to take it orally (and also as nose drops several times a day)."

"I have to say that within a few days I felt so good. The constant pain is gone and I can actually think really clearly. I made the comment to my husband the other day that I lived so long with Sinus that I didn't realise how good it feels to be without pain and to feel really clear headed. I just want to say thank you for a truely amazing product and one that won't be detrimental to my health in the long term." TA

Tooth root canal infection
"I was told by my dentist that there was absolutely no cure or treatment for the very bad Root Canal Infection that was constantly oozing pus through the gum."

"I took 10mls twice a day of Colloidal Silver and put a pad of cotton wool soaked in Silver on my infected gum over a few nights. The result was a very rapid healing. Within days all signs of infection disappeared. Every few months I repeat this to keep it under control. It is quite remarkable." JR

Traveller's Diarrhoea

"My work as a marine engineer takes me all over the world, and many out of the way places, where 'Traveller's Diarrhoea' is endemic. I have found in every case, every time, that the minute I feel any kind of stomach cramp or discomfort after a meal, I take 25mls (5 teaspoons) of Colloidal Silver in a glass of water and the usual diarrhoea is averted." JGN

Mastitis

"I had returned from an overseas trip and found I was developing a new round of Mastitis on the plane. By the time I got home I was pretty sick and the Mastitis was advancing."

"I had no antibiotics until two days later. By then I was very ill and the antibiotics were not helping. I think I had had them so many times in the past months they were not working."

"My Dad arrived with a new thing, Colloidal Silver. I tried it. Next morning my Mastitis was completely gone. My 104 degree fever was gone. My breast was not red or swollen."

"My baby had not been nursing well at all during this bout of mastitis. I had to use hot compresses to get even one drop of milk from my right breast. But by the next morning my milk was free flowing and I felt great." Jeana, USA

Contact lens eye infection

"The most remarkable change I have noticed is in using the undiluted Colloidal Silver drops as an eye rinse twice daily. I use an eye dropper and put in several drops morning and evening. The first two days my eyes stung slightly, and in the morning I woke up with a slight discharge in the corner of my eyes. After that, my eyes which were always bloodshot from years of adverse reaction to wearing Contact Lenses with harsh chemicals, and having eye infections which prescriptions didn't solve, were snowy white! I didn't think that a 46 year old lady could have snowy white eyes after the problems I had. They are like a healthy young child's."

"I decided to store my lenses in Colloidal Silver. I use half of the soaking solution and half distilled water. To that I add 3 drops of Colloidal Silver and shake. To my amazement the solution is so gentle I don't have sore eyes any more." BW

Sore throat

"I was suffering the worst infection in my throat I have ever

51

had, and the infection kept getting worse. I went to our local health store and bought a bottle of Colloidal Silver. I used it directly in my mouth and within 20 to 30 minutes I felt the difference. I was amazed how fast it attacked the infection and destroyed it. It really does work."

Well readers, that's information from letters I have received, letters I have seen on the Internet, and letters from Sota Instruments health newsletter. Go to the Internet and a search engine, type in 'colloidal silver heal' and you will get thousands of answers.

Before I finish with Colloidal Silver let me explain some other uses of Colloidal Silver.

Breast Cancer

It is estimated (USA figures) that one in four women will develop Breast Cancer in their lifetime.

I know of two women who claim to have healed themselves of Breast Cancer with Colloidal Silver. They were both diagnosed by biopsy. After the diagnosis they took two teaspoons of Colloidal Silver daily until their surgery. One took a homemade product, the other a Silver protein product. In both cases the second biopsy of the removed breast tissue and lymph nodes were cancer free!

What we don't know is, will Colloidal Silver work this well for all Breast Cancer patients? Dr R.O. Becker in his book **"The Body Electric"** found that in the presence of Silver, cancer cells reverted back to normal cells.

Also, Cancer research scientist Dr Gary Smith stated, *"When Silver is present, the Cancer cells dedifferentiate* (normalise) *and the body is restored."* Also, *"I suspect a Silver deficiency is possibly one of the main reasons Cancer exists and is increasing at such a rapid rate."*

Try this experiment

Go into your garden; pick two flowers off the same plant. Put one in a water filled vase, leave the other lying on the bench for about eight hours. By this time it will be quite limp.

Fill a vase with Colloidal Silver. Cut the stem a little shorter and drop it in. Next day it will be standing upright. More than that, despite being half dead and in extreme stress, it will not
52

only recover, but will then outlive the flower that was placed in water immediately.

This should help you to believe there is a life-giving quality to the Silver colloid.

Hundreds of other uses

Mildew-free paint

If you are using a water-based paint, and are painting a side of a building that sees little, or any sun in the winter, mix about 5% of high strength ppm Colloidal Silver in with the paint. Mildew will not find a home on your paint. To make high strength Colloidal Silver run your generator four times longer than normal.

Vegetables or Flowers

When planting out, water your plants with Colloidal Silver.

Use it as a fungicide to spray your plants and fruit trees to keep them free from blight or bacterial pests or moulds.

I came across this testimonial from a hydroponic grower:

"Since using Colloidal Silver on our hydroponic lettuce we have been able to control aphids, and there has not been any sign of caterpillars in the lettuce or broccoli. Being very allergic to pesticides I am grateful that I can now spray regularly with Colloidal Silver with no ill effects to myself, and be able to provide my customers with produce that is not full of insecticides."

Spray it on your body

- To remove acne.
- To remove itchiness between legs, or around anus from haemorrhoids.
- Immediately on a wasp or bee Sting to greatly reduce swelling or pain.
- Into your mouth to remove toothache, ulcers and bad breath (drink some as well).
- Under arms to remove sweaty bacterial odours.
- Onto feet and into shoes for athlete's foot.
- Into eyes and ears to kill infections.
- Soak contact lens or dentures.
- Onto baby's skin to eliminate nappy rash, measles, chicken pox, rashes.
- Also use for psoriasis, boils, eczema and scratches.

In your home

- Spray your benches and cutting board to remove all bacteria.
- Into jam before sealing.
- If you have been sold milk that has a use by date only three days ahead, you can at least double its life by adding a teaspoon of Colloidal Silver and stirring or shaking.
- Spray your refrigerator to prevent smells.
- Wipe your telephone receivers and head phones.
- Spray combs and hairbrushes.
- Sterilise tooth brushes and dentures.
- Wipe toilet seats.
- In your shower spray to keep mildew off walls

These are but a few of the hundreds of uses you will find for your body and around your home for Colloidal Silver.

Purifying water

To purify water for storage, add 2 teaspoons of Colloidal Silver per litre. If the water is thought to contain harmful bacteria, double this to 4 teaspoons.

Prevention of spoilage

To prevent the fermentation or growth of bacteria in canned foods or fruit juices, add 2 teaspoons of Colloidal Silver per litre

One thing not to do

If you have a septic tank for sewage treatment, do not ever empty a large amount of Colloidal Silver down your waste water or it may kill the bacteria in your septic tank.

Well readers, learn from what I have written and from what people have told me.

Other products being called Colloidal Silver

At the time of writing, there were four products available in America being called Colloidal Silver. No doubt some of these others will soon be available here.

The first product is the one I make, **Pure Colloidal Silver**.

The second is called **Mild Silver Protein.** This product chemically binds microscopic particles of Silver to a protein molecule. It is usually found in concentrations of 20-40 ppm. Its appearance may be transparent, clear, or amber.

The third product is **Silver Salts.** This is made chemically or electro-chemically and contains a form of silver that dissolves in water. Concentrations range between 50-500 ppm. Appearance is transparent-clear. The silver particles carry a positive charge, but almost invariably there are other elements and compounds beside silver.

The fourth is sometimes referred to as **Powdered Silver.** This product was developed by the Russians and is made when a pure silver wire is rapidly disintegrated by a high voltage electrical discharge similar to an old photo-flash bulb. The microscopic silver dust is collected and either dissolved in water, or added to salves and creams for topical use. Concentrations range from 100-500 ppm.

Hit or miss

To one degree or another, all these products work as a broad spectrum germicide because they all contain microscopic particles of silver.

That said, it is important to understand a number of things. All these products are not colloidal suspensions of silver. They do not behave the same, either in the body or laboratory tests. Effectiveness and dosage varies from product to product, and from batch to batch, as does quality. They are not all uniformly safe and non-toxic.

Best to make your own

Increasingly, more and more people are finding the

tremendous advantages to health and pocket by using Colloidal Silver, but by far the best way to control quality is to make your own. By doing this you will end up with Pure Colloidal Silver, which is what this book is about.

Will Colloidal Silver eliminate all illnesses of the human body?

While Silver will kill hundreds of pathogens, it does not mean Colloidal Silver will eliminate all the illnesses they cause in the human body. Certainly in the test tube they all die, but they have many refuges in the human body where they can hide from Silver colloids in the blood.

Shingles is a good example. Colloidal Silver taken internally will reduce a shingles infection from being worryingly painful to barely a tingle. But if you remove the Silver colloid from your diet the original condition will return.

Colloidal Silver is the best medicine anyone can take for a host of problems, but the biggest obstacle to people treating themselves is the lack of information in the public domain as to how to use it effectively in a given situation.

Before giving Colloidal Silver a totally clean bill of health in the USA in 1936, the FDA (Federal Drug Agency) tested it very extensively. It has on record all the different doses and concentrations needed to kill different micro-organisms and the exposure times for a total kill.

Why Pharmaceutical companies don't like Colloidal Silver

Pharmaceutical companies cannot patent Colloidal Silver, therefore they have no control over its price to build in massive profit margins. So naturally they would never put up ten million dollars to research just how good it is. They also know that if knowledge of cheap Colloidal Silver reaches the wider public domain, their profits will plummet.

If the FDA were to release its records of how good Colloidal Silver is, the drug companies would probably find a reason to claim the findings were unsubstantiated and insist that the FDA test Colloidal Silver with the same rigour they are supposed to use in testing their drugs.

This would take about ten years and cost the taxpayers over

a billion dollars to prove to the FDA what they already know. If that happened I have not the slightest doubt that the drug companies, with the help of politicians would win the battle to control Colloidal Silver.

The facts are that the whole medical system of the western world is captive to the politics of big money and big drug manufacturers.

The FDA has never spent the public's tax dollars discovering anything important, and then published their findings for the public at large. Especially when it involved something that was powerful, safe, and inexpensive and that the public could make for themselves.

Obviously, empowering the population to be self-reliant and frugal in relation to their own health care is not a high priority to the Federal Drug Agency.

Do-it-yourself health care may not be worse

The OTA (Office of Technology Assessment) is a government department in the USA that studies and analyses technological procedures.

Their report on medicine in the early 1990's stated that almost 80% of medical procedures don't work and have little scientific basis, and that most people just heal, despite medical mistakes.

For example – a Harvard university study of heart patients found that 84% of people told by their doctor they needed bypass surgery, in fact did not need it!

Worse than that, three separate studies have since found that people do not live longer because of bypass surgery. So why do it? Well consider this – heart surgeons in America gross 28 million dollars a day on heart surgery.

Many people, are coming to the conclusion we have to look after ourselves. Keeping healthy and treating ourselves may be a far cheaper and more reliable method.

The blackout in medical schools about Colloidal Silver

I am astounded by the almost total lack of knowledge among the medical profession about the deadly efficiency of Colloidal Silver against the whole spectrum of illnesses caused by bacteria, fungi and viruses.

Ask almost any nurse, doctor, pharmacist, or veterinarian about Colloidal Silver. Most of them know nothing or very little about it!

So the suppression starts right at the top. Can you think of a reason why? There is a very simple explanation, MONEY!

Consider this – if a bottle of Colloidal Silver could cure Colds, Shingles, Whooping Cough, Sore Throats, Athletes Foot and all of the hundreds of illnesses caused by bacteria, fungi, or viruses within a few hours, or a day or two, how many people would pay to visit doctors?

The pharmacist would have a savage drop in income too. Hardly anyone would be coming in with prescriptions from the

59

doctor. And don't forget the pharmaceutical industry. If hospitals could make their own Colloidal Silver on the premises so cheaply they could swab the floors with it, to whom would the drug barons sell their unneeded products?"

What motivates most doctors?

A survey of medical students in an American Medical School in early 1980 discovered that 84% of them were not training to be doctors because they wanted to do something helpful for mankind, but because they considered they would be in a very highly paid and prestigious job.

One can only wonder, after the years of training by example from our political leaders to *'look after number one'* would any different result be found in New Zealand?

A money-sucking scandal

What needs to be done in our society to stop this money sucking of the public purse, not to mention the years of unnecessary pain and suffering by people with Shingles and similar ailments.

In my opinion nothing less than a commission of inquiry into all aspects of modern medicine, and some very valid reasons why such a totally harmless substance such as Colloidal Silver should not be used for the benefit of humanity.

The best health insurance

Colloidal Silver has extraordinary capabilities and hundreds of uses, but without public experiments we will never know the best way to use it in a given situation.

Colloidal Silver can enhance the health of you and your family in hundreds of ways. The best health insurance you will ever buy is to purchase a Silver generator and make Colloidal Silver for yourself. And to do it before private manufacture is banned and the only people who will be able to sell and prescribe it will be drug companies and doctors.

Colloidal Silver is not a panacea

You cannot drink unlimited alcohol, smoke unlimited cigarettes, eat copious fatty meals, and expect to heal your health problems with Colloidal Silver alone. Your choice of lifestyle is and always will be a major factor in good health.

Despite increasingly favourable feedback from health researchers around the world about overcoming all types of so called incurable disorders by use of the dirt-cheap method of Colloidal Silver, not one government Health Department in the world appears to be investing any money whatsoever into formal research. The facts seem to be, as far as they are concerned, *'over 65, better dead.'*

In this book I have laid down facts of happenings to myself, and friends, and told stories from other researchers of their successes. If you wish to take charge of your own health it is now entirely up to you.

Enjoy good health from this four way attack

1. Eat a healthy diet of unprocessed foods, and supplement with trace minerals like Selenium, Zinc, Magnesium, Boron, etc, that are lacking in our soils. (If you don't believe trace minerals are lacking in our soils, speak to any New Zealand farmer.)

2. Ingest Colloidal Silver.

3. Do about an hour's exercise a day.

4. Reach out and help others.

PART TWO OF THIS BOOK
Read the facts and decide for yourself

Before I go into the second part of this book, I feel it is essential for you to know the qualifications of the people I am talking about.

For myself, I am just a 77 year old retired farmer. Left school at 14 years of age. No qualifications except a School Proficiency Certificate I obtained at the age of 12.

But this book is not about me. I am just putting before you, facts, happenings, researches, and results of some highly qualified and successful men who have helped people otherwise condemned to death or suffering by a stubbornly orthodox medical profession. A profession that is living in the dark ages as far as many new treatments for illnesses are concerned.

It seems almost inconceivable, that in a so called modern state such as America, that police with drawn guns could invade doctor's surgeries, seize records, and lay charges against them to remove their licences to practice medicine because they dared to heal 'incurable diseases' with unorthodox treatments. None of which treatments used any of the numerous poisonous substances sold by drug companies and approved by the FDA.

But in America and Canada, even today it still happens.

Who is Doctor Hans Nieper 1928-1999?

Dr Hans Nieper was a famous medical researcher and has been called a medical Einstein. His father was also a doctor, in Hanover, Germany and he taught his son from the earliest age never to accept tradition as fact, and to always explore for better treatments.

Dr Hans Nieper followed his father's footsteps and trained to become a doctor in Freiburg University, where he paid particular attention to physics and medicine.

In 1952 while studying for his thesis, he discovered that the body's immune system could become corrupted and actually

62

consume and neutralise parts of the body's defence system against Tuberculosis.

To suggest a living organism would consume part of itself was not an easy way to find favour with the medical profession in those days, especially when orthodox medicine scoffed at such a suggestion. But he argued his case with such logic before a panel of the best pathologists in Germany that he gained his doctorate with top honours.

It was the first time an auto-immune system had been demonstrated to exist, and it reinforced a position Dr Hans Nieper was to hold throughout his lifetime. That the treatment of disease must commence at a cellular level!

He soon became heavily involved with Cancer research. At that time everyone was seeking a quick cure, a 'magic bullet.'

There was no magic bullet

The most promising approach was using derivatives of mustard gas called Malines. These were nasty poisons for cancer cells and with severe side effects for other cells, but showed some promise with Leukemia and Lymphomas.

It was at Freiburg University that Dr Hans Nieper received his first shock regarding the suppression of medical information. The research team he was with were getting ready to publish some research facts stating that while Malines showed some promise, they were toxic and very slow acting.

However the head of the research department ordered them not to publish. They found out later he was applying for another job at a more prestigious university, and was worried that he might not get the job if his team reported little effective progress.

The only effective way to fight Cancer

After spending a further 18 years on Cancer research and studying the body cells inability to recognise Cancer cells, Dr Hans Nieper came to the conclusion that the only effective way to fight Cancer was to stimulate the cell's own immune system, or to repair the damaged DNA that allowed the uncontrolled growth of cells.

He had also discovered the value of dietary minerals in helping stimulate the immune system, and in protecting the integrity and DNA of healthy cells.

At this time, in the mid 1960's, the most prestigious Cancer research faculty in the world was the Sloan Kettering Institute in America where the world's best researchers were working.

Dr Hans Nieper's brilliance resulted in him being invited to work in Sloan Kettering. He was a gifted researcher and his knowledge of Cancer treatment was extensive and advanced, so he was more like a professor than a researcher.

It was an open secret that one of Sloan Kettering's executives had earlier sent his mother to Dr Nieper's clinic in Germany for treatment.

Apricot Stones

Although Dr Nieper had done no research on it himself, he had heard of a promising derivative of apricot stones called Laetrile or Vitamin B17. He was also aware that the AMA (American Medical Association) had ridiculed it and denounced any doctors who were experimenting with it as 'quacks.'

Therefore he was amazed after arriving at Sloan Kettering to hear their Cancer researchers tell him that the most promising substance they had yet found to fight Cancer was Laetrile!

Every other substance they had so far researched, damaged other cells and the whole immune system, whereas Laetrile only targeted Cancer cells and did no damage to any other cells.

An experiment of my own

Let me digress a little here regarding apricot stones. After long research over many decades, medical researchers had found two groups of people in the world among which Cancer was extremely rare. One group was the Hunzas in the Himalayas, and the other the Eskimos.

The Hunzas had great longevity, many lived to over 100 years of age. They did not eat refined western foods, and apricots in season were a large part of their diet.

The difference between the Hunzas and Europeans was that when we eat an apricot we toss away the stone, whereas the Hunzas crack every stone and eat the flesh and the kernel.

Eskimos don't grow apricots, but they do eat a berry that has the same Cancer-protecting property and enzyme as apricot stones.

Nevertheless, in the 1970's the AMA denounced Laetrile as a quack medicine and refused to allow doctors or anyone to manufacture or possess it.

Our own NZ Health Department and doctors sheepishly followed the same bleating, *"Don't eat apricot stones, they will kill you!"*

Just how poisonous are apricot stones?

Well, knowing the history of the AMA and the quackery and gangsterism involved in its early leaders, and the habit of its leaders even today of having the opposite of inquiring minds, I was extremely suspicious of their howlings and decided to test for myself just how poisonous apricot stones really were.

I had an apricot tree in my garden and saved every stone. I started off eating five kernels a day for seven days.

Nothing happened!

Ten a day for a week. Nothing!

Fifteen a day for a week. Nothing!

Twenty a day. Nothing!

At 25 apricot stones a day, I felt a little squirmish and ended the experiment.

Apricot stones poisonous? Not unless you eat bags of them!

Laetrile an effective anti-Cancer agent

We must remember that the researchers and other genuine doctors around the world were not using apricot stones, but a derivative from them, of which Dr Nieper said a few years before he died, *"Laetrile (Laevomandelonitrile) extracted from apricot pits is one of the most powerful anti-Cancer substances found. It is a non-toxic compound comprised of glucose, cyanic acid, and benzaldehyde. Cancer cells produce rhodanase, an enzyme, at their membrane surface. The Laetrile molecule is split by the rhodanase at the Cancer site and releases cyanic acid, which is highly toxic to Cancer cells but does no harm to other cells. This is the mechanism by which Laetrile is an effective anti-Cancer agent."*

Don't report the truth, report what we pay you to say!

Now the Sloan Kettering Institute employed a publicity agent to tell the public all the benefits of the latest drugs they were researching and to encourage people to donate support for research. His name was Dr Ralph Moss.

But when word leaked out that Sloan Kettering researchers had found simple apricot stones held a promising substance to treat cancer, the Sloan Kettering top bosses immediately issued a statement saying they had, *"researched Laetrile and found it valueless."*

Sloan Kettering's senior researcher, Japanese Doctor of Science, Dr Sugiura, refused to accept this distortion of facts. He stated, *"I write what I see. Laetrile is a good palliative Cancer drug."* Dr Sugiura was hounded and ridiculed for contradicting his employers.

Dr Ralph Moss also refused to support the lie and was sacked *'for failing to carry out his basic responsibilities.'* Dr Moss later clarified this by stating, *"That meant he had refused to lie when his boss had told him to."*

Dr Ralph Moss later wrote a number of books, among them, **'Questioning Chemotherapy', 'The Cancer Industry'** and **'Cancer Therapy'.**

No money in apricot stones

Dr Nieper's opinion of the sudden about-face by Sloan Kettering was that the drug companies were unable to patent apricot stones, and that the big financial sponsors of the Institute had told them to experiment only on drugs they could patent, manufacture, and make a profit from.

Dr Sugiura returned to Japan where he refined a helpful Cancer drug from the active ingredient in apricot kernels.

Electricity and the human body

Very early in his training as a physicist, Dr Hans Nieper realised that doctors not only had to have the knowledge to diagnose an illness, but also to understand why it occurred. The only way to do that was to understand the basic structure of cells.

In gaining such knowledge during a very productive lifetime

Dr Nieper realised that the human body was an electro-magnetic organism, and that magnetic fields had an effect on our health.

He also pondered the fact that the human heart, with such a low pumping pressure could not push freshly oxygenated blood throughout our bodies in seven minutes, unless veins were almost frictionless. He eventually concluded that like magnetic trains whose wheels never touched the rails, our blood must be delivered throughout our bodies by a similar magnetic mechanism.

Negatively charged minerals

He and other researchers also discovered that every healthy cell carries a positive charge of electricity. In the field of magnetism, like repels like and they discovered that even though cells need nourishment from trace element minerals, positively charged minerals had difficulty in entering cells.

It is also interesting to note that in 1998, medical research showed that the first line of defence for cell protection is an electrical discharge at the invaders.

Take note of this article in the French magazine "Science et Vie" September 1998, which quotes researchers from the Geneva University Hospital in Switzerland.

I have translated it into layman's language. *"White cells kill bacteria and pathogenic fungi by electrocuting them. As soon as white cell receptors detect the presence of a microbe, they send a signal to sleeping enzymes, which become activated. They load up with electrons and are transported to the area for defensive action. Then the enzymes eject an electronic flux of charged oxygen molecules and the microbe dies."*

Oratates, Arginates and Aspartates

Brilliant work by physicists in the 1960's found a way to place a negative charge on mineral salts of Calcium, Magnesium, Potassium, Zinc, Lithium, Selenium and others. They were named Oratates, Arginates and Aspartates, or AEP for short.

They have revolutionised the treatment of Multiple Sclerosis, Diabetes, Osteoporosis, Asthma, Cancer, and Retina Eye Disorders to name just a few.

These substances were later licensed as a medicine by the

German health authorities under the name of Vitamin Mi, for the treatment of Multiple Sclerosis.

In Germany there is a hospital licensed for alternative medicine called the Paracelsus Hospital of Alternate Medicine. It is located at Lake Silbersee in Hanover. It was here that Dr Nieper worked most of his lifetime.

Here's what Dr Nieper wrote about Diabetes

Dr Nieper began using these negatively charged minerals on his patients and found they had many other extremely useful applications besides Multiple Sclerosis. This is what he writes after more than thirty years of observation and experience.

"The application of Calcium Arginates and Magnesium Arginates belongs to the most positive experiences in my entire life. The blood sugar drops in a most spectacular way. In one case the administration of Calcium and Magnesium Arginate dropped the morning glucose reading from 300 down to 134 with no change in diet."

He also writes regarding Diabetes Type 2: *"I think we made a major breakthrough in the control of this most vicious disease."*

Dishwashing detergent and Diabetes

Dr Nieper believes that one of the causative factors of Diabetes Type 2 is contact with residual detergent on dishes. He suggests that only Citric Acid be used in dishwashers and for hand washing dishes.

Diabetic Kidney and Retina failure prevented by Calcium EAP

He also states *"The kidneys are the organs most endangered by Diabetes on a long term basis. It is a diabetic's fate to frequently suffer kidney failure and be connected to a dialysis machine. We have observed in 24 years of administering Calcium EAP that Diabetic Retinopathy will practically not occur."*

"Having collaborated with several Ophthalmologists in Germany and the USA we are now certain that this therapy is extremely effective in retaining the function of the retina. The kidneys also are protected in a manner unimaginable up to now."

High Blood Pressure and Varicose Veins almost entirely eliminated

"During the last 30 years we have been able to observe that for patients taking Calcium and Magnesium AEP, the development of Thrombosis, Circulation problems, High Blood Pressure, and the progression of Varicose Veins is almost entirely eliminated."

Asthma and MS success with Calcium EAP

"Now we almost have no Asthma patients left, especially none of younger or middle age."

"While formerly one third of all MS patients would die of lost nerve functions, and another one third of increased tendency to bone fractures, and the last one third of kidney failure, only two patients out of 2,200 did this."

Any hospitals in NZ found out about it yet?

The odd doctor up with the play in Germany, Italy, and America now uses these substances, but monopoly drug companies do not make them, nor seem to want anyone to hear about them. I doubt if we will hear of them in New Zealand for a decade or two yet.

If you give yourself Aids via your own lust, or accidentally get Aids from a bad blood transfusion, politicians will use our taxes to pay for drugs at over $10,000 a year to keep you alive for five, ten, maybe fifteen years.

But if you ask politicians to allow doctors to prescribe modern natural substances, proven to be non toxic, with no side effects, and having the ability to cure, they will not even listen. They prefer to be guided by the steeped-in-drug-company-orthodoxy, doctor-priesthood, not modern doctors of physics and medicine.

Yet over a period of 25 years, perhaps millions of people who could have been healed have died. Why? Because to adopt methods like Dr Hans Nieper's would cause enormous financial loss to those who manufacture expensive cancer treatment equipment, or high-priced drugs to sell to cancer victims who will not be cured.

69

Not to mention the enormous loss of income to doctors, hospitals, undertakers, and all incomes derived from the 'Cancer Industry' which in America involves approximately some 20 billion dollars yearly.

Governments around the Western world only subsidise and promote the use of drugs, not natural substances for alleviating illnesses. So people who choose to be treated with non-toxic products like minerals, vitamins and amino acids either have to pay the full cost themselves, which most cannot afford without taxpayer help, or put up with, in many cases, useless, painful orthodox treatments.

People suffering from cancer may find the following interesting

This is from an article published in the German magazine "Raum und Zeit." I quote: *"Even though large specialised hospitals have not acknowledged the fact, it is nevertheless true that extraordinarily expensive Chemotherapy and Radiology are without a doubt a failure. The internationally recognised Oncologist, Dr Hans Nieper from Hanover, Germany reports in this article, "... a promising therapeutic possibility in conquering cancer, namely the application of active substances from plants (and insects) for the repair of genetic information which got lost in cancer cells."*

Note. The two substances are Dionaea, made from the Venus Fly trap plant, and Irrododial, made from ants.

Breast cancer self-healed 30 years ago

Regarding the repair of the body's DNA, consider this 30 year old German report. *"In 1973 a so called 'spontaneous healing' of advanced Breast Cancer was witnessed in the Silbersee Hospital in Hanover, Germany. The healing process was very dramatic, and with the help of money donated by the Volkswagen Car Company the cancer patient was given extensive tests to try and determine the cause."*

"The tests revealed that the cause of the rapid disappearance of wide-spread cancer metastasis throughout the bones of the patient appeared to have its foundation <u>in the ability of the body to repair a derailed genetic system in the cancer cells, not the usual 'immune system' response</u>, as with people responding to

bacterial or viral infection."

Dr Hans Nieper's books

As mentioned earlier, Dr Hans Nieper is now regarded by top medical researchers around the world as a medical Einstein.

He has written two books that I know of, which anyone who would like to find out about modern medical healing needs to read. The most recent one, written in 1999, the year he died is called **"The Curious Man: The Life and Works of Dr. Hans Nieper."** It deals with the medical life and work of Dr Nieper in which he explains methods and substances for treating Multiple Sclerosis, Diabetes, Cancers, etc.

Besides being a doctor and a scientist, he wrote over 300 papers on space, magnetism, electrical fields, and alternative sources of energy. In 1972 he published a paper on the **"Shielding Theory of Gravity"** dealing with vast untapped fields of energy around us. NBS the big American TV newscaster did a half hour program on some of the 'impossible' machines that were not supposed to work, but did.

Despite being swamped by popular demand for a repeat of the program, it never again appeared on TV. Such programs make oil suppliers throw wobblies and threaten to withhold advertising.

The other book, which I believe he wrote in the 1970's is called **"Dr. Nieper's Revolution in Technology, Medicine and Society."** It deals mainly with alternative energy sources, and also a little on medicine. Both these books and his medical substances are available in New Zealand.

Other interesting health findings

Here are some more findings of interest.

Kidney stones – a human pearl?

Researchers looking for a cause as to why kidney stones form, were surprised when splitting one open to find tiny live 'nano-bacteria' in the very centre. They now theorise that these ultra-tiny bacteria (one nano is one thousand-millionth of a metre) irritate the kidney, which like a pearl oyster covers the irritant with a secretion of mineral, and like a pearl it just grows. These incredibly small bacteria thrive in urine.

Ten years ago, if any researcher suggested there were such things as nano-bacteria they would have been ridiculed, because the experts had worked out that no bacteria would ever be found under 250 nanometres in size, because it would be impossible for such creatures to function. Well, in 1998 three researchers claimed to have found some nano-bacteria just 11 nanometres in size.

I remember when I first learned about atoms at school, I was taught they only had three parts. Now scientists have discovered, by smashing atoms to bits, that there are hundreds of parts to an atom.

Dr Phillip Hylemon of US Virginia Medical College suggests that the common bacteria Clostridia and Eubacteria may play a similar role in the foundation of gallstones.

A cause of Alzheimers?

Let's have a look at that terrible brain disorder of the aged, Alzheimer's. This mind-destroying disease is being studied at the Wayne State School of Medicine in New York.

Doctors there reported in 1998 that they had isolated the bacteria Chalmydia Pneumonia in the brains of 27 out of 29 people who had died with Alzheimer's, and had only found this bacteria in the brains of one of 18 people who had died of other causes.

Magnets help many people

It is interesting to note in recent years that patents have been taken out by physicists or doctors regarding the use of powerful magnetic fields to heal various ailments.

These include three patents for the killing of micro-organisms, five patents for killing cancer, one to fuse bone, one to modify cells, one to reduce serum glucose, and one to carry out cleansing of pathogens from the blood.

Magnetism has been considered a health aid by many people for hundreds of years. Recently a magnetic blanket has appeared on New Zealand markets with a 100 day trial and money-back guarantee if not helpful. They are proven to help many people.

Why the Health Industries are worried about real cures

Right around the world, vast quantities of money are spent yearly on Cancer, Aids, Hepatitis C, Lupus, etc.

What would happen if you could treat and cure these diseases in your own home without drugs or medical treatment? All people in the 'Health Industry' would suffer a drastic fall in income, as they would have hardly any customers.

But the major reason why these health inventions will never see the light of day is that we tend to elect dumb politicians who cannot understand that people are in the main not needed to create wealth, machines can do it far more tirelessly and efficiently.

They also reason that the last thing a nation can afford is to have too many of its elderly living past 65. They will have to pay out too much money in pensions.

But they have little to fear, few people will read this book and other books like it. And of those that do, only about 10% of them will action what they have read.

For those of you who do want to keep well, and wish to take action to stay that way for a few more years, the first thing to do is to take some Colloidal Silver every day. You can buy a Silver generator to do that for around $200. That will quieten down a lot of pathogens in your body.

Aspartame, food additive number 951

If you have friends or relations with Multiple Sclerosis, Lupus, Hepatitis, Cancer, Aids, Shingles, Epstein Barr, Paget's Disease, Diabetes and a number of other so called incurable diseases, then you may well be interested in this information.

Early this year 2000, Nancy Markle spent three days lecturing at the World Environmental Conference on Aspartame, marketed as 'NutraSweet,' 'Equals,' and 'Spoonful' and commonly used as a sweetener in diet soft drinks.

The keynote speaker at this conference spoke of an epidemic of Multiple Sclerosis and Lupus, and how they did not know what toxin was causing this to be rampant across the USA. Here is what Nancy reports:

"I explained that I was there to lecture on exactly that subject."

"When the temperature of Aspartame exceeds 86°F, the wood alcohol in Aspartame converts to Formaldehyde, and then to Formic Acid (another name for Methyl Alcohol or Methanol) *which in turn causes metabolic acidosis* (acid blood)."

Mimics MS and triggers Lupus

"The Methanol toxicity mimics Multiple Sclerosis. Thus people were being diagnosed with having Multiple Sclerosis in error. Multiple Sclerosis is not a death sentence, but Methanol toxicity is."

"In the case of Lupus, we are finding it is becoming almost as rampant as Multiple Sclerosis, especially among Diet Coke and Diet Pepsi drinkers."

"Also with Methanol toxicity the victims usually drink three to four 12 oz cans a day, some even more.

"In the case of Lupus, which is triggered by Aspartame, the victim generally does not know that Aspartame is the culprit. The victim therefore continues using it, aggravating the Lupus to such a degree that sometimes it becomes life threatening. When we get people off the Aspartame, those with systemic Lupus generally become asymptomatic (their symptoms disappear)."

"Unfortunately we cannot reverse this disease. On the other hand, those diagnosed with Multiple Sclerosis, when in fact they are suffering from Methanol toxicity, generally recover when off Aspartame."

Tinnitus

She had also seen cases where victims' vision and hearing had returned. This also applied in a case of Tinnitus.

During a visit to a hospice, a nurse told her that six of her friends who were heavy Diet Coke addicts had been diagnosed with Multiple Sclerosis. This is beyond coincidence.

Aspartame converts to Formaldehyde in the retina of the eye, causing blindness. Formaldehyde is a deadly poison and is grouped in the same class of drugs as Cyanide and Arsenic. It just takes longer to kill, but it is killing and causing all kinds of neurological problems. It changes the brain's chemistry. It has been known to cause severe seizures and also causes birth defects.

Aspartame makes you fat, average weight loss when off Aspartame – 8 kgs

Imagine what it does to patients suffering from Parkinson's Disease. There is absolutely no reason to use it. It is not a diet product. It makes you crave carbohydrates and will make you fat.

Dr Roberts, a diabetic specialist and world expert on Aspartame poisoning stated that when he got patients off Aspartame their average weight loss was 19 pounds (8½ kg).

He said, *"Formaldehyde stores in the fat cells, particularly hips and thighs. It is especially deadly for diabetics, blinding them with diabetic retinopathy. It keeps the blood sugar level out of control, causing them to go into a coma. Unfortunately many have died."*

"People were telling us at the American Conference of Physicians that they had relatives who had switched from Saccharin to an Aspartame product, and how those relatives had eventually gone into a coma. Their doctors could not get the blood sugar levels under control. Patients suffered acute memory loss and eventually coma and death."

Kills your brain neurons, escalates Alzheimer's

Dr Roberts also tells how Aspartame is escalating Alzheimer's disease. *"A hospice nurse told me that women are being admitted with Alzheimer's disease at 30 years of age."*

Dr Russell Blaylock, a neurosurgeon said, *"The ingredients in Aspartame eventually stimulate the neurons in the brain to death."*

Aspartame is sold in over 90 countries. Some 5000 food products now contain it. Monsanto, the manufacturers know how deadly it is, just as the tobacco companies knew about nicotine.

Monsanto funds the American Diabetic Association and the Conference of the American College of Physicians.

The New York Times, November 15, 1996 ran an article on how the American Diabetic Association takes money from the food industry to endorse their products. Therefore they cannot criticise any additives or tell of their link to Monsanto.

Desert Storm War mysterious illness

During the Desert Storm War some years ago, thousands of pallets of diet drinks were shipped to Saudi Arabia and sat in the hot sun for months. Remember that heat over 86°F liberates the Methanol from the Aspartame. Thirsty troops slaked their thirst with this poison. No wonder so many came home with indefinable illnesses, all of which are identifiable with Aspartame poisoning.

Dr Roberts says that consuming Aspartame at the time of conception can cause birth defects. The Phenylalanine concentrates in the placenta and can cause mental retardation. It can also cause brain tumours.

When Dr Episto was lecturing on Aspartame, a neurosurgeon in the audience said that, *"When we remove brain tumours we often find high levels of Aspartame in them."*

Well readers I had to prune it a little but left in all the essentials.

Look out for these symptoms

Just a reminder, some popular Vitamin C tablets contain Aspartame. So do most chewing gums.

If you use a lot of it in your food and drink, watch out for the following symptoms, Fibromyalgia, Spasms, Shooting pains, Numbness in your legs, Cramps, Vertigo, Dizziness, Headaches, Tinnitus, Joint pain, Depression, Anxiety attacks, Slurred speech, Blurred vision.

Any of these may be a sign of Aspartame poisoning.

Stop using it!

Other Books By Zealand Publishing House

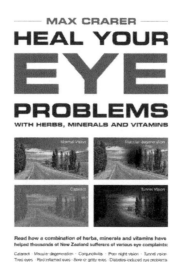

MAX CRARER

HEAL YOUR EYE PROBLEMS

WITH HERBS, MINERALS AND VITAMINS

Read how a combination of herbs, minerals and vitamins have helped thousands of New Zealand sufferers of various eye complaints:

Cataract · Macular degeneration · Conjunctivitis · Poor night vision · Tunnel vision Tired eyes · Red inflamed eyes · Sore or gritty eyes · Diabetes-induced eye problems

Prevent and Heal your eye disorders naturally. Max Crarer's unique New Zealand Book will show you how This highly interesting NZ Book "Heal your Eye problems with Herbs, Minerals and Vitamins was written by retired farmer Max Crarer of Wairoa while in his mid 70's. There appears to be no other book like it in the world.

It tells a true story of how several years earlier he accidentally healed his Glaucoma (of 12 years standing)

Max was well known to listeners of Radio Pacific and shared his story with them before writing his book

Thousands of New Zealanders with eye complaints helped by Max

Following his own healing, Max researched other eye natural healings from eye researchers all over the world.

78

Since then, through his own experience and numerous personal experiences of others, including his Radio Pacific listeners, he discovered combinations of herbs, minerals and vitamins that have helped thousands of NZ sufferers of various eye complaints. These herbs, minerals and vitamins are all available from NZ health shops. His book tells you all that he has learned.

Prevent and heal cataracts

Herbs minerals and vitamins have also been found to prevent and heal cataracts (cloudiness in the lens). Max's combinations normally clear a lens of a cataract naturally in six months.

Glaucoma and Macular Degeneration have responded

Max does not claim that his herb, mineral and vitamin recommendations will heal every eye condition. However, when his practical advice is acted on in good faith, most eye conditions, even some considered incurable by many Ophthalmologists, successfully respond.

Glaucoma and Macular Degeneration have long been considered incurable. However Max reveals herb, mineral and vitamin combinations that have healed both these disorders.

Simple tests for Glaucoma and Macular

Max's book also contains simple home tests for early detection of Glaucoma and Macular Degeneration that you can do yourself at home.

Treatable eye disorders

All the following eye problems are treated in this book: **Glaucoma, Cataracts, Macular degeneration, Tunnel vision, Conjunctivitis, Discomfort in strong light, Poor night vision, Red inflamed eyes, Sore eyes, Tired eyes, Drooping eyelids** and **Diabetes-induced eye problems.**

Easy-to-read, highly interesting book

Max's highly interesting, useful, and boldly written book is easy-to-read and reasonably priced.

As a bonus, it also contains a section on low-cost and little known cures for some common ailments, such as: **Arthritis, High blood pressure, Stomach ulcers, Sagging skin, Kidney stones, Gall stones, Fluid retention** and **Repetitive Strain Injury.**

The Most Authoritative Guide to Health on the Market

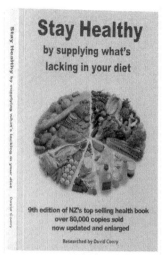

This best seller with over 65,000 sales in Australia and New Zealand, by David Coory continues to be one of New Zealand's top selling health books and for a very good reason...

This book tells you exactly how to ensure that your body gets the full Recommended Daily Intake (RDI) of essential vitamins and minerals from food and supplements that your body needs to stay active and healthy.

It is difficult to obtain all of the vitamins and minerals that our bodies need in the average diet, something that can lead to worrying and often dangerous deficiencies. For instance, New Zealanders have the lowest levels of the vitally important mineral selenium, and many are also deficient in calcium. Every country has their unique deficiniecies. This book tells you how to overcome this problem and recommends the foods that can address this as well as the minerals and vitamins and their functions.

David's thorough research and candid writing style make this an easy read full of useful information about health. Every Doctor should have to read this as a part of their training to become a doctor.

80

19137253R00046

Printed in Great Britain
by Amazon